W9-BIZ-788

Eating for Two

Also by Mary Abbott Hess and Anne Elise Hunt

Pickles & Ice Cream: The Complete Guide to Nutrition During Pregnancy

A Healthy Head Start: The Worry Free Guide to Feeding Young Children

By Mary Abbott Hess

The Art of Cooking for the Diabetic (coauthor)

EATING *for* TWO

The Complete Guide to Nutrition During Pregnancy

MARY ABBOTT HESS,
L.H.D., M.S., R.D.

ANNE ELISE HUNT

MACMILLAN • USA

Macmillan General Reference
A Simon & Schuster Macmillan Company
1633 Broadway
New York, NY 10019-6785

Copyright © 1994 by Stephen M. Pollan and Mark Levine

All rights reserved. No part of this book may be reproduced or transmitted in any form or by any means, electronic or mechanical, including photocopying, recording, or by any information storage and retrieval system, without permission in writing from the Publisher.

MACMILLAN is a registered trademark of Macmillan, Inc.

Illustrated by Keith Taylor
Book design by Jennifer Dossin

Library of Congress Cataloging-in Publication-Data

Hess, Mary Abbott.
Eating for two: the complete guide to nutrition during pregnancy/
Mary Abbot Hess, Anne Elise Hunt.
p. cm.
Includes bibliographic references and index
ISBN 0-02-065441-3
1. Pregnancy—Nutritional aspects. I. Hunt, Anne Elise.
II. Title.
RG559.h45 1992
618.2'4—dc20 91–47161 CIP

10 9 8 7

Printed in the United States of America

Contents

Foreword

Prenatal care—the early, regular, and continuing medical assessment and care of the pregnant woman—was introduced during the early twentieth century. It has been the principal factor responsible for the marked improvement in healthy pregnancy and childbirth over the past fifty years. Prenatal care has several aspects, but there would be little argument that nutrition is among the most important. Put another way, what a woman eats during pregnancy is a potent determinant of her own health and that of succeeding generations.

One of the more encouraging of modern trends is the interest today's mother-to-be has in understanding pregnancy and childbirth and in taking an active role in her own care. Mary Abbott Hess and Anne Elise Hunt's *Eating for Two: The Complete Guide to Nutrition During Pregnancy* is of great value in this regard. It is comprehensive, thorough, and balanced in reviewing the intricacies and complexities of this most marvelous of physiologic processes. Further, it is absolutely up-to-date, drawing heavily on the 1990 report of the Institute of Medicine's Food and Nutrition Board's Committee on Nutritional Status During Pregnancy and Lactation. This report was commissioned by the U.S. Department of Health and Human Services. Having had the privilege of chairing that committee, I take special pleasure in seeing the committee's work translated into practical and consumer-oriented advice so quickly and so accurately.

Eating for Two extends beyond the strict boundaries of nutrition, encompassing a number of other aspects of prenatal care. While the emphasis is on normal pregnancy, as it should be, the book also provides insight into some of the more common problems and abnormalities that can arise.

Coming from a long-standing and highly productive collaboration between a nutritionist and a writer, this book presents the best of science in an extraordinarily readable style. An earlier version, under a different title, enjoyed substantial popularity. I recommend it to many of my own patients, as well as to a lovely woman pregnant with what was to become my first grandchild. The new version is even better, though I don't see how it can produce a better grandchild.

ROY M. PITKIN, M.D.
Professor and Chairman
Department of Obstetrics and Gynecology
UCLA School of Medicine

Preface

About ten years ago, we wrote a book about nutrition during pregnancy. The book is out of print, and we wanted to write another on the subject. Little did we realize when we started our project that so much had changed in a relatively short period of time! There are new recommendations about weight gain, protein requirements, vegetarian meal-planning, supplements, food safety, and medications. Foods with sugar and fat substitutes, foods reduced in fat and sodium, foods fiber-enriched or calcium-spiked forced us to expand our traditional food lists.

"Older" mothers are now mainstream, and research studies unavailable only a decade ago are responding to their increased numbers and special needs. Exercising women now have guidelines to ensure safe but effective workout programs both before and after delivery. Many more women are working through pregnancy and returning to work after giving birth. Life-styles have changed, and so have cooking and eating habits.

This book is for every woman, no matter what her eating habits. It's for you who don't eat it if it doesn't come in a bag or a box, who eat out several times a week, load up the shopping cart with frozen entrees and containers from the salad bar and the deli, regularly order pizza and Chinese food delivered, and indulge in rich ice cream and then righteously drink diet soda. This book is for you who buy fresh fruit and vegetables, eat yogurt and bran flakes, and read labels to cut salt and fat and cholesterol. It is for all of you who *now* want to eat what is best to have a healthy baby.

This book is also for physicians, nurses, registered dietitians, and others who work with pregnant women. In preparation, we reviewed hundreds of articles in current journals of obstetrics, nursing, and nutrition, and we read background material in many textbooks. We drew from newspapers and magazines, attended lectures and presentations, conducted telephone interviews with professionals, and listened to tapes on the subject. We reviewed the background information from the committee that issued the 1989 Recommended Dietary Allowances. We eagerly awaited the publication of the report of the Committee on Nutritional Status During Pregnancy and Lactation, and incorporated its findings when it was released in 1990. We worked together on the book until Anne, who does not have a technical background, could understand it, and Mary, who is a registered dietitian and former professor, said it was accurate. Because we also wanted to create a book that would relate to the life-styles of today's women, we shared our own experiences and those of our families, friends, and colleagues.

Then we sent the manuscript to experts who counsel pregnant women, conduct research, and write for professionals about prenatal nutrition. We incorporated their changes and suggestions and considered their many thoughtful, probing questions. We want to thank them for their talent, their time, and their support: Pat L. Bull, R.N., I.B.C.L.C., certified lactation consultant, The Breastfeeding Connection, Naperville, Illinois; Roy M. Pitkin, M.D., Department of Obstetrics and Gynecology and chair of the Committee on Nutritional Status During Pregnancy and Lactation, School of Medicine, University of California at Los Angeles; Julie Scheier, R.D., Prentice Women's Hospital, Chicago, Illinois; Madeleine Sigman, Ph.D., R.D., Department of Food Science, Pennsylvania State University, State College, Pennsylvania; Carol West Suitor, D.Sc., R.D., Bethesda, Maryland; Bonnie S. Worthington-Roberts, Ph.D., chief nutritionist, Child Development Center; professor of Nutritional Sciences, University of Washington, Seattle, Washington.

We wrote this book because pregnant women want and deserve to have sound information to guide food choices that will promote their own health and that of their baby.

To our readers, we send wishes for a wonderful, healthy pregnancy and a perfect baby.

1
Welcome to My Womb

Pregnancy is an almost sacred responsibility. When you carry a child, you are forging a link in the chain of life—a link between past and future generations. But the goal is not merely to carry on the species. Parents also want to give birth to a baby who will be able to thrive and reach its full potential as a healthy, happy human being.

Short-term efforts to improve the outcome of pregnancy have long-term implications not only for the child but for the parents as well. A child who is born strong and healthy has fewer illnesses throughout life than a child who is born very small or with detectable problems at birth. Healthy babies grow up to do better in school and have fewer behavioral problems than infants with health problems at birth.

Every pregnancy is unique and influenced by thousands of variables. Some variables, like genetics or the mother's age, are not controllable. But maternal nutrition is a matter of personal choice. So are drug and alcohol use and smoking.

Until recently, the concept of the fetus as a parasite whose needs take priority over the needs of the host (or in this case, hostess) was widely accepted. In fact, while some changes do take place in pregnancy to help protect the fetus, nature actually favors the mother's needs more than the baby's. When a mother-to-be is not eating an adequate diet, she and her baby compete for nutrition. In the long run, neither of them gets sufficient nourishment.

This book is about healthy babies *and* healthy mothers. If the quality and quantity of the mother's diet are adequate, both before conception and during pregnancy, fewer complications are likely during pregnancy and labor, and the mother has a greater chance of giving birth to a larger, healthier baby. In addition, the mother's recovery is faster, and breast-feeding is more likely to be successful.

THE NUTRITIONAL LIFELINE

An amazing thing happens when an embryo attaches itself to a woman's uterus. Nature "hides" the embryo, first by suppressing the cells that reject foreign bodies (such as skin grafts). Then, the embryo is surrounded by tightly-packed cells that form a protective barrier.

Maternal and fetal blood never mix. The fetus is dependent upon the mother but maintains its own systems. An "exchange" takes place in the *placenta.* The fetus is connected to the placenta by the *umbilical cord.* The cord contains one vein that carries oxygen- and nutrient-containing blood to the fetus, and two arteries that return waste products and carbon dioxide to the placenta. There are no nerves in the umbilical cord, which is why the baby feels no pain when the cord is cut at birth. The umbilical vein and arteries project into the placenta in little rootlike structures called *villi.*

Maternal blood flows into the placenta through arteries in the placental wall. The blood pools around the fetal villi. Here the critical transfers take place. While the placenta was once thought to act as a *barrier* to substances in the mother's blood that could be harmful, now we know that size and chemical structure, not potential toxicity, dictate what goes through the placenta. It is more accurate to describe the placenta as a filtering system or sieve than a protective barrier.

Some substances pass readily from the mother to the fetus by a process called *diffusion.* If, for instance, the mother takes megadoses of fat-soluble vitamins A or D, the vitamin will seep, or "diffuse," from the mother's blood into the fetal bloodstream until the vitamin concentrations are equal. Levels that may not be harmful to an adult woman can endanger a developing baby.

Most proteins do not cross the placenta, since they are too large to be absorbed by the villi. Instead, there is an exchange of amino acids, the building blocks of protein. From

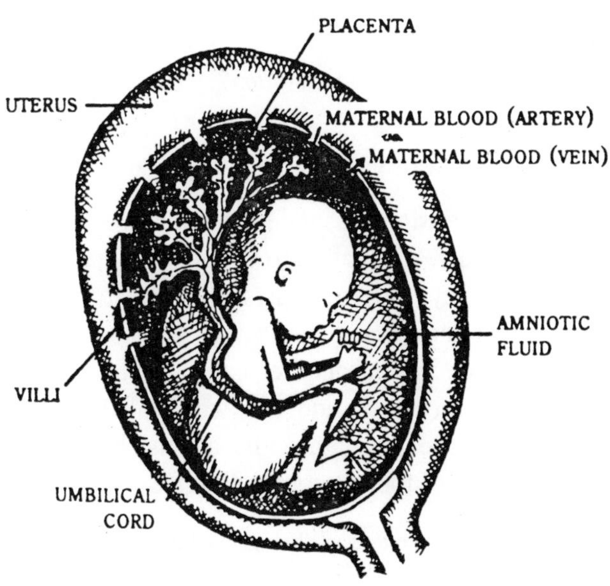

amino acids, the fetus can make the various proteins it needs for growth and development.

One protein, however, called immunoglobulin IgG, does cross the placenta intact. IgG gives the baby the mother's antibodies that resist infectious disease—kind of a prenatal vaccination. IgG continues to protect the baby for the first six to nine months after birth (202).*

Most substances in the fetal bloodstream that are not used are carried back through the umbilical arteries, pass through the placenta, and return to the maternal bloodstream to be processed or excreted. Other substances, such as vitamin C, are converted in the fetus into complex forms or become trapped in the fetus and cannot pass back through the cell walls of the villi. Thus, potentially harmful concentrations can build up in the fetus.

Unfortunately, many drugs, chemicals, alcohol, and medications can pass through the placenta and, as part of the fetal bloodstream, influence cell development. We will discuss these substances in detail in chapter 7, "Playing It Safe."

Delivering Nutrients on Schedule

The average full-term pregnancy lasts 280 days, or approximately nine months. The baby grows and develops during all phases of pregnancy, different parts at different times. Too many or too few nutrients, especially as organs are forming or bones and blood are building, can result in fewer cells or imperfectly formed cells. In addition, what you eat will influence the size of the placenta and maternal blood supply, essential elements of the nutrient delivery system.

* Numbers given in parentheses throughout the book correspond to the numbered entries of the Bibliography.

YOUR BABY'S GROWTH

TIME	DEVELOPMENT
First Trimester	Vital need for good nutrition to support growth of maternal tissue and development of fetal internal organs, limbs, and sense organs
Fertilization	Implantation in uterus
7 days	Embryo is the size of the head of a pin
	Primitive circulation between placenta and embryo is established
4 wks (1 mo)	Beginning of eyes, ears, spine, digestive tract, limbs, brain, nervous system, and organs
Second Trimester	Crucial time for refinement of physical structures
	Respiratory and cardiovascular systems are inadequately developed for life outside of mother's body
	Mother's mineral intake important for developing strong bones and blood in fetus
16 wks (4 mos)	Scalp hair appears
	Motor activity begins
	Digestive system develops; heart muscle develops; kidneys are in place
	Weight, 3–4 ounces; length, about 7 inches
Third Trimester	Fetus doubles in size in this trimester
	Nutrients and calories are vital to development of the baby and preservation of maternal stores

TIME	DEVELOPMENT
	Transfer of minerals to baby's body to calcify bones and to build iron reserves in liver for the first few months of life
28 wks (7 mos)	Body developing fat; nails appear; lungs and eyes develop
	Weight now about 3 pounds; length, 14 to 17 inches
32 wks (8 mos)	Fetal weight is increasing rapidly
	Calcification of bones in fingers and toes; teeth are developing
	Transfer of iron to baby's liver to protect against anemia in early infancy
	Taste sense is present; developing reflexes and behavior patterns
	Weight almost 4 pounds; length, 16½ to 18 inches
36 wks (9 mos)	Skin smooths as fat forms under it
	Lungs are fully developed; metabolic system is developing to support life after birth
	Sex organs are well developed
	Fetus is able to sustain life outside womb
	Weight almost 5 pounds
40 wks (birth)	Skin smooth
	Insulation of brain begins; brain cells continue to develop
	Weight about 7 pounds if it's a girl and 7½ pounds if it's a boy; length, about 20 inches

BIRTH WEIGHT

Bigger, Better Babies

Adequate birth weight is critical to getting your child off to a good start in life. Full-term babies weighing seven pounds or more* have several important advantages over full-term babies weighing five and a half pounds or less. Babies of adequate birth weight

- Have fewer physical handicaps
- Are less likely to have birth defects
- Have a lower rate of infant mortality
- Are less likely to be mentally retarded
- Are more likely to have higher IQs
- Suffer fewer serious illnesses during childhood
- Have fewer hearing and visual disorders
- Are less likely to have respiratory and other infectious diseases
- Have fewer behavioral problems
- Are more mature and better able to handle environmental stress
- Have a head start both physically and mentally over their smaller peers who may never catch up.

Mother's Weight and Gain

The mother's prepregnancy weight and the total weight gained during pregnancy are, except for the length of preg-

* Data on American infants show that average birth weights range from six pounds 10 ounces to eight pounds thirteen ounces. In this book, when we refer to a "normal seven-pound baby," we are referring to this range of weights. Genetic potential, including the parents' sizes, will influence the baby's weight; thus, some "normal" babies may not fall within this range.

nancy, the two most important factors in determining birth weight.

As soon as you've announced to your friends and family that you are expecting a baby, you will begin to receive advice and counsel—especially about how much weight you should gain. Some say more weight is better; others say less. Even doctors don't agree.

Advice about how much weight a woman should gain during pregnancy has changed considerably over the years. Women once tried to keep weight gain to a minimum in order to create smaller babies and thus ensure an easier delivery. Then, in the 1950s and 1960s, studies began to show how adequate weight gain affected healthy fetal development.

In 1970, the Food and Nutrition Board's Committee on Maternal Nutrition set the desirable average gain at between twenty and twenty-five pounds (129). The American College of Obstetricians and Gynecologists and the American Dietetic Association concurred. Still, some physicians continued to support restricting weight gain to twenty pounds or less.

Today, you can find advocates from both extremes: Some physicians argue in favor of limiting weight gain, while at the other end of the spectrum is a school of thought that prescribes no limits, insisting that "eating to appetite" during pregnancy, even if it results in excessive gain, is the "natural" and right way. The consensus of scientific thought today is between the extremes—twenty-five to thirty-five pounds for a healthy woman who is not under- or overweight when she becomes pregnant (172).

It takes fifteen to twenty pounds of "maternal equipment" to produce a seven- or eight-pound baby. To begin with, you can't have a baby without a placenta (which represents about 5 percent of total weight gain) and amniotic fluid (which makes up 6 percent of weight gain). Your blood volume jumps 50 percent—more if the baby is larger—accounting for another four or five pounds.

Fluid retention varies greatly from woman to woman. Some women hold as much as eleven pounds of body water (172). The uterus, enlarged breasts, and "maternal stores" contribute the other pounds. Maternal stores is necessary fat accumulation—nature's calorie reserve for pregnancy and lactation. Underweight women with poorly developed maternal stores have trouble supplying enough energy to support rapid fetal growth during the last trimester and they are under more stress during labor and delivery.

If you already have plenty of fat stored in your abdomen and thighs, you may want to assume that you can use what's already there. But nature can't be fooled. Stored body fat is not the stuff of which sound babies are made (197). If you are overweight, you will need to work closely with your doctor or a registered dietitian during pregnancy. While you don't want to gain more than necessary, you do want to be sure to gain enough. A gain of less than fifteen pounds can jeopardize fetal growth and development of other essential components of pregnancy—a smaller placenta will limit the amount of nutrients your baby receives; a reduced blood volume can deprive the baby of oxygen.

It is startling to find that 25 percent of women giving birth in 1980 in the United States gained less than twenty-one pounds (203), and 12 percent gained less than sixteen pounds. To a large extent, these statistics reflect socioeconomic factors and drug abuse. Some women, however, did not gain weight because they had poor eating habits, were severely underweight before pregnancy, skipped meals, or dieted during pregnancy. Many women who work at maintaining a slim figure have a hard time accepting their weight gain; women who are overweight are similarly concerned about gaining weight; working women may feel pregnancy interferes with "looking professional." Whatever the reason, inadequate weight increases the risk of having a small baby.

Recommendations for Weight Gain

How much weight you should gain during pregnancy depends to some extent on your prepregnancy weight. Are you normal for your height, overweight, or underweight? Use the table below to categorize your prepregnant weight so you can then get a general idea of how much you'll need to gain during pregnancy. You can use the information in this book to discuss specific weight gain with your doctor.

WEIGHT-FOR-HEIGHT TABLE FOR NONPREGNANT WOMEN

HEIGHT W/OUT SHOES	STANDARD WEIGHT	UNDERWEIGHT (BELOW)	OVERWEIGHT	VERY OVERWEIGHT (ABOVE)
4′9″	105–126	104	127–137	138
4′10″	107–130	106	131–141	142
4′11″	109–132	108	133–143	144
5′	111–134	110	135–145	146
5′1″	114–137	113	138–149	150
5′2″	116–141	115	142–153	154
5′3″	119–144	118	145–156	157
5′4″	122–147	121	148–160	161

HEIGHT W/OUT SHOES	STANDARD WEIGHT	UNDERWEIGHT (BELOW)	OVERWEIGHT	VERY OVERWEIGHT (ABOVE)
5′5″	124–150	123	151–163	164
5′6″	127–154	126	155–167	168
5′7″	130–157	129	158–171	172
5′8″	132–160	131	161–174	175
5′9″	135–164	134	165–178	179
5′10″	141–170	140	171–185	186
5′11″	142–172	141	173–187	188
6′	143–174	142	175–189	190
6′1″	146–177	145	178–192	193

SOURCE: Adapted from 1983 Metropolitan Life Tables

BABY-BUILDING FOR THE NORMAL-WEIGHT WOMAN

A healthy, normal-weight woman should expect to gain twenty-five to thirty-five pounds during pregnancy to produce a healthy, normal-sized baby (172). This recommendation of the Institute of Medicine's Subcommittee on Nutritional Status and Weight Gain During Pregnancy is higher than previous recommendations.

The subcommittee's premise is that the higher gain reduces the risk of delivering a baby that is small for the length of time it has been carried. The range reflects the variations of normal gain experienced by individual women. Young women tend to gain more than older women; first-time mothers gain more than those who have had other children; small-framed women gain more than larger-framed women; tall women gain more than short women; and African-American and Hispanic women gain less than white women.

BABY-BUILDING FOR THE UNDERWEIGHT WOMAN

If you were very underweight when you became pregnant, you are at risk of having a baby weighing less than five and a half pounds if you gain less than twenty-eight pounds during pregnancy. To reduce this risk, underweight women should gain twenty-eight to forty pounds during pregnancy (172).

An underweight body will compete with the developing baby for nourishment. If the fetus does not get enough nutrients from the food you eat, it will draw upon your body. When your own stores are inadequate, your body resists such deprivation, and the baby's growth is limited.

Underweight women are typically advised to make every effort before and during pregnancy to achieve their ideal body weight in addition to gaining extra pounds for pregnancy. Dr. Myron Winick, a well-known authority on nutrition in pregnancy, questions whether standards used to determine ideal weights for underweight women are realistic. Advising a very thin woman to gain to 120 percent of her ideal weight (which may be over forty-five pounds) by the time she delivers may be unreasonable and, if the amount is very great, may even be undesirable, Dr. Winick contends. Experts agree that every effort should be made to encourage an underweight woman to get closer to her desirable weight before conception so that she and her child do not compete for nutrients during pregnancy. Note: Dr. Winick and many other health professionals use the term "ideal" weight when describing the best possible weight-for-height range. We think the term "desirable" sounds more reasonable and achievable.

If you are underweight, the first question to ask is, Why? Do you like the way you look when you are thin? Is your weight the result of poor eating habits? Do you come from a family with "thin genes"? Do you have food intolerances or other conditions that limit your food choices? Do you smoke? Does drinking or taking drugs interfere with normal eating? Are you a serious athlete with very little fat tissue? As you examine your reasons, consider what you might change in light of your goal for pregnancy: a healthy baby.

The nutrition chapters in this book will be especially important for you to read because it is likely that your nutritional status can be improved. It is hard to change set patterns, but the effect will have lifetime implications for your child.

On the other hand, you may enjoy the added weight. A friend of ours told us, "At five feet eight inches and 117 pounds, I had for years been referred to as having a 'Care package look.' My gynecologist said, 'Eat what you like,' and I did. Fifty pounds later, I had breasts for the first time and an astounding belly, which from the rear was not noticeable but from the side I looked like a pregnant thermometer. I was voluptuous for the first time in my life and loved it. I enjoyed eating and delivered an eight-pound baby boy. Within six weeks, I was again 117 pounds."

BABY-BUILDING FOR THE OVERWEIGHT WOMAN

The best time to lose excess weight is before you become pregnant. Dieting to avoid weight gain during pregnancy can be dangerous to your unborn child. Broken-down fat cells are a poor source of energy for building a baby. When body fat is burned, ketones (a form of acid) are released. Ketones can be detected in urine samples; your doctor may test for the presence of ketones if your rate of weight gain is below the normal range. The hazards of burning fat for energy are discussed more in chapter 4 (202).

Your goal now is to gain fifteen to twenty-five pounds. The

target weight gain for very overweight women is fifteen pounds. (We use the terms *very overweight* or *severely overweight* because we don't like the term *obese* used in the medical literature.) Severely overweight women are more likely to develop hypertension and diabetes during pregnancy than women weighing less, but there are no data showing whether a gain of more than fifteen pounds increases that risk (197). And, although healthy babies are born to very overweight women who gain less than the recommended amount, a gain of less than fifteen pounds is not recommended (172).

An overweight body doesn't necessarily mean an adequately nourished body. In fact, many overweight women are undernourished. Babies need more than fat to grow on. Body fat can be the result of excessive calories from fat, sugar, or alcohol—all poor sources of vitamins and minerals. Body fat cannot be changed or converted to protein and other nutrients the baby needs for proper development. If you are overweight, you will need to make food choices that provide the essential nutrients (without excessive calories) you and your baby need. If you are very overweight, work closely with a registered dietitian or your doctor throughout your pregnancy to monitor the amount and rate of weight gain.

Being severely overweight increases the risks of gestational diabetes and hypertension, which in turn can influence fetal growth and health. Severely overweight women are more likely to have complications during labor and delivery. It is dangerous to the developing fetus to diet during pregnancy. You will still have your weight problem after delivery, but pregnancy is *not* the time for a very calorie-restricted diet. For overweight women, the focus should be on *quality* rather than quantity of food. Good eating habits established during pregnancy can become the foundation of long-term weight management.

BABY-BUILDING FOR THE WOMAN CARRYING TWINS

There are no studies in current medical literature that provide specific recommendations for weight gain for women who are carrying twins and were under- or overweight before pregnancy. However, women who gain inadequate weight increase the likelihood of preterm delivery and smaller babies (172).

Women who carry twins should aim at a total weight gain of thirty-five to forty-five pounds (172). To deliver babies that are at least five pounds each, in a gestation period that is generally two to three weeks shorter than for a woman carrying a single child, the mother should try to gain about one and a half pounds per week in the second and third trimester (172). Beginning about week sixteen, the weight-gain standard with twins swings up sharply, in contrast to the single-baby standard (202).

How Much Is Too Much?

Further weight gain beyond recommended amounts does not mean you will have a bigger baby. Basically, you are adding to yourself—not to your baby. The trick here is pacing the gain. You can't gain the full amount in the first six months and then try not to gain more. If you are gaining too much weight, or at too rapid a rate, it's time to talk to your doctor or a registered dietitian.

A large weight gain may make labor more difficult and prolong the second stage of labor. Women carrying a single baby who gain more than forty-six pounds are more likely to have a cesarean delivery or one that necessitates the use of forceps (172). There are, however, women who gain as much as fifty or sixty pounds, experience normal labor and delivery, and have healthy children. Although large weight gain does not affect the development of the baby, the fewest risks and complications are associated with a weight gain within the recommended ranges.

The Subcommittee on Nutritional Status and Weight Gain During Pregnancy contends that the trend toward larger babies does not account for the remarkable increase in cesarean deliveries in recent years (172). The subcommittee's major concern is that very high maternal weight gain may lead to postpartum obesity. And obesity is a risk factor for heart disease, stroke, diabetes, hypertension, and other problems.

Until recently, the main concern about high weight gain was toxemia, now called pregnancy-induced hypertension (PIH). A study of a large group of women who gained more than thirty pounds during pregnancy showed that while 9 percent developed PIH, 91 percent did not (129). PIH is also associated with *low* weight gains (172), inadequate medical care, age (under twenty, over thirty-five), and chronic hypertension (202).

If you find yourself eating too much and gaining too quickly, take steps to cut calories without losing nutrients.

Pattern for Growth

The pattern and rate of gain seen by charting weight monthly and then weekly indicates whether you and your baby are progressing normally. If you suddenly put on two to five pounds in one week, or fail to gain at recommended rates in the third trimester, you should seek prompt medical attention (172).

CUT CALORIES, NOT NUTRIENTS

Do

Use lowfat milk and dairy products
Choose lean cuts of meat
Avoid fried foods and rich desserts
Eat vegetables and fruit instead of high-calorie snack foods
Drink no-cal water when you're thirsty
Use reduced-calorie salad dressings, mayonnaise, and margarine

Do Not

Skip meals
Cut out cereals, whole grains, or starchy vegetables
Drink fewer than 4 glasses of lowfat milk (or equivalent) each day
Severely restrict salt
Use diuretics

During the first few months, you *feel* but don't necessarily *see* changes. More than thirty hormones are busily preparing your body for the months ahead. The uterus is growing and blood volume begins to expand. At this point, the fetus weighs only a few ounces. While your weight may not be shooting up, you *will* notice changes in your body—goodbye waistline!

Your weight gain may be minimal, especially if you suffer from the nausea so common to early pregnancy. But don't

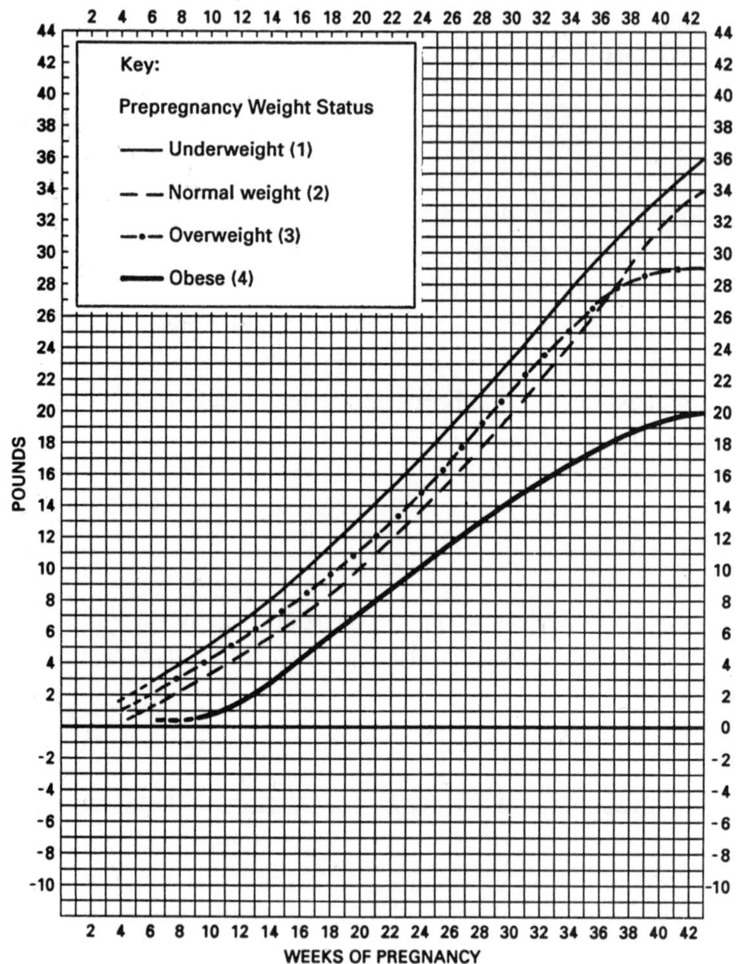

RECOMMENDED WEIGHT GAIN PATTERNS

This chart shows the recommended weight gain pattern for women who at conception are underweight (1), normal weight (2), overweight (3), and obese (4).

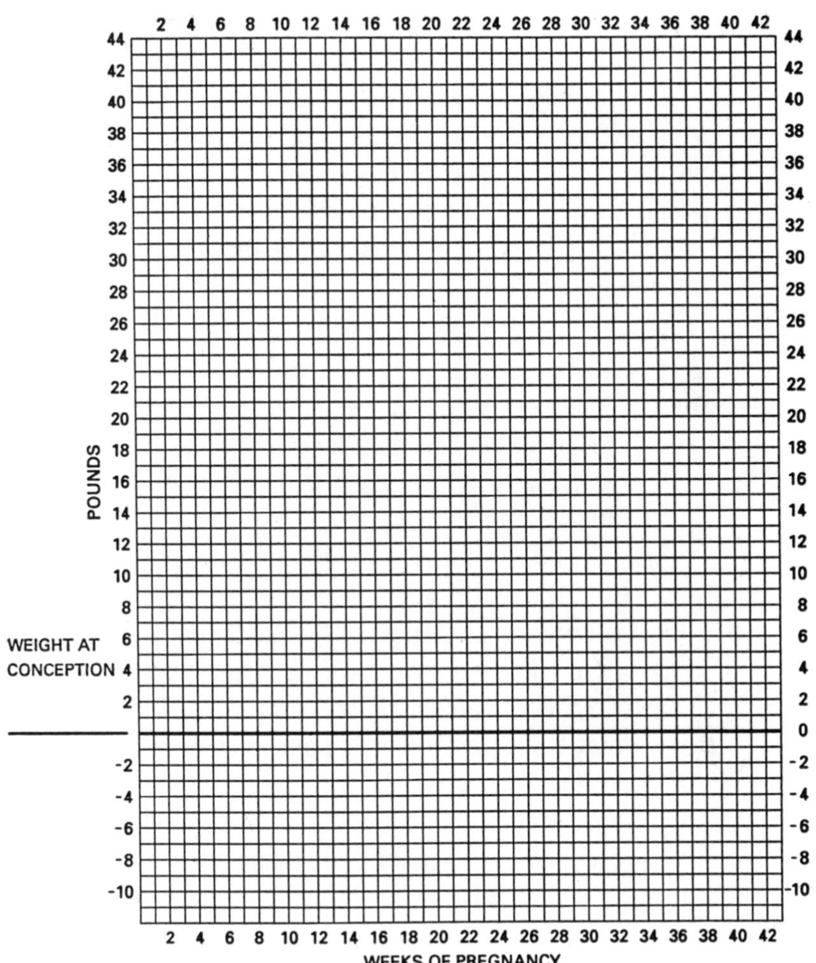

CHART YOUR WEIGHT GAIN

Write your weight at conception in the space provided. Each week, place a dot to indicate your weight gain (or loss) since the previous week. Every week, weigh yourself on the same day, just after you get up in the morning and before you get dressed. Connect the dots to chart your weight gain.

worry. There is little association between weight gain during the first trimester and the birth weight of the baby.

All of a sudden, usually about the three-month mark, the baby begins to shoot up (or out, we should say). From this point on, weight gain for normal-weight women is about a pound a week. For a woman carrying twins, the goal is one and a half pounds per week during the second and third trimesters (172).

Normal-weight women carrying their first child can expect to gain at the following rates:

- 0–10 weeks: about ½ pound per month
- 10–20 weeks: about ¾ pound per week
- 20–30 weeks: about 1 pound per week
- 30–40 weeks: about ¾ pound per week

Underweight women should attempt to gain:

- first trimester: about 2 pounds per month
- second trimester: about 6 pounds per month
- third trimester: about 5 pounds per month

Overweight women should try to gain:

- first trimester: about ¾ pound per month
- second trimester: about ¾ pound per week
- third trimester: about ½ pound per week

It is important to remember that these amounts, like most estimates in this book, are averages. Some women gain more, others less, and are still perfectly normal. But if you are consistently far from the average, talk to your doctor about the reasons.

Hello Baby, Goodbye Weight

In the week following their baby's birth, most women lose the majority of the weight they gained during pregnancy.

Another four to six pounds usually disappears by the time the baby is six weeks old. But it can take as much as a year and a half to get back to feeling energetic and well-toned. Some maternal weight added during pregnancy may be retained permanently (172). On average, a woman retains about 2.2 pounds after each pregnancy. Those who gain more when they are pregnant tend to retain more after they deliver, simply because they have stored additional fat.

Even if you are close to your prepregnancy weight 6 weeks after delivery, you may struggle with leftover fat that doesn't want to go away. (172, 129) Women who have been told that breast-feeding will give them back their prematernal figure may become discouraged, and some give up nursing in order to begin dieting. Weight-loss for nursing mothers is discussed on page 273.

A good program of exercise can help restore prepregnancy figures. Unless you have a cesarean section, you can begin a regular exercise program six weeks after giving birth, when the uterus has returned to normal size and position. Programs for new mothers include low-impact aerobics, light calisthenics, and stretching exercises. Follow the guidelines of the American College of Obstetricians and Gynecologists (ACOG), outlined in chapter 2, and use ACOG's excellent postpartum exercise tape.

PRE-CONCEPTION PLANNING

The very best time to prepare for pregnancy is before conception. Current research suggests that early cell divisions, those that happen shortly after conception before a women knows she is pregnant, are particularly important. Preparing an environment with a blood supply rich in nutrients and without alcohol or chemicals from drugs gives your baby the very best start.

If possible, begin planning for pregnancy several months ahead.

- Select your obstetrician.
- If you use oral contraceptives, stop taking them for at least two months before you try to get pregnant.
- Have a complete physical, including a blood analysis that will indicate your iron status.
- Be tested for rubella and have the monovalent rubella vaccine, if necessary, right after your period to be sure that you are not pregnant when you are inoculated. Wait until you have had another period before you try to conceive.
- Get yourself as near as possible to desirable weight for your height.
- Discuss use of vitamin-mineral supplements and prescribed medications with your doctor.
- If you smoke, drink alcohol, or use recreational drugs, *stop now!*

Reducing the Risks During Pregnancy

While pregnancy is a normal condition, it is also a special time—a time for extra care. Under most circumstances, babies grow and flourish if given proper nurturing. But every mother-to-be should know that there are substances and situations that create physiologic stress and can interfere with normal development.

You are at risk of developing problems during pregnancy if you

- Are significantly underweight or overweight
- Are on a weight-loss diet
- Are younger than age seventeen
- Have a great deal of emotional stress
- Eat no meat, poultry, fish, eggs, or dairy foods
- Smoke
- Consume alcoholic beverages
- Take large quantities of vitamin-mineral supplements
- Are under treatment for preexisting medical problems
- Take prescription drugs that are not safe during pregnancy
- Use nonprescription drugs, such as aspirin, that are not safe during pregnancy
- Use "recreational" drugs (marijuana, cocaine, etc.)
- Have a history of obstetric problems

You can take action to reduce most of the risk factors. This book can help you improve your eating habits; we hope it will inspire you to make life-style changes and give up potentially harmful habits. If you need nutrition counseling, your doctor may provide it or can refer you to a registered dietitian, a nutrition clinic at the hospital, a public health nutritionist, or a nutritionist with a community-based program.

Special women's clinics provide many helpful services, including stress management and support groups for pregnant women. Hospitals, health clubs, YWCAs, and community centers have exercise classes for pregnant women. But be careful about exercise services; some may be run by individuals who are not qualified and who do not follow the ACOG guidelines. Substance abuse counselors are available through women's clinics, hospitals, or the March of Dimes Birth Defects Foundation, and are listed in the yellow pages of your local telephone directory.

We hope that this book will help you know what questions to ask, encourage you to ask the tough questions, and motivate you to make changes to help your baby reach its full potential.

We wrote this book to provide basic information needed to make informed choices about nutrition during pregnancy. No book can replace the services of a physician. Good medical care is essential to both you and your baby.

2

Assessing Your Nutritional Status

Pregnant women differ in many ways. Experts make recommendations that can be applied broadly to the population as a whole. But to be useful, generalities must be tailored for individual use. You may rightly ask, What about *me* and *my* baby? This book will help you find the answers you need.

The Preliminary Inventory that follows will help you identify personal characteristics and habits that can influence your pregnancy. We will discuss the implications of this profile in the chapters that follow. Throughout the book, we have included short questionnaires to help you evaluate your own habits, spot your strengths, and determine areas that warrant change. Short quizzes along the way will uncover myths about pregnancy, put to rest some unnecessary concerns, and stir up other concerns that can make a difference.

If you are in the planning stage, and hope to become pregnant in the near future, the Preliminary Inventory will identify nutritional needs you can start working on right now. But regardless of where you are in your pregnancy, it's never too late to improve your diet and health habits. The environment you create within your body is much more important to your baby than the nursery in which it will spend its first months.

PRELIMINARY INVENTORY

Age 25 Height 5'3" Due date 7th Apr

Ethnic origin Asian

Weight before pregnancy 83 pounds

Are you underweight, overweight, or normal weight? (See table, pages 10–11.) UW

Describe your feelings about weight gain during pregnancy. I feel that I should gain weight in my stomach area. Moreover, I feel that I have began to gain weight in small doses. I am scared about it.

Describe any health problems you have. No health problem till now. But now a days I get a little bit of stomach ace and also my legs hurt.

Are you under a physician's care for these problems? no.

Describe any nutrition-related illness you have had in the past, such as anemia, anorexia, or bulimia. none

List prescription drugs you take.____Advil. (none)____

Do you take vitamin-mineral supplements?____no____

If yes, were they prescribed by a doctor?____–____

Describe type of supplement and amount you take.____– NA____

List nonprescription drugs you take (aspirin, cold capsules, diuretics, etc.).________

Are you now taking birth-control pills, or were you prior to becoming pregnant?____no____

Do you have a history of heavy menstrual flow?____yes____

Are you carrying more than one baby?________

Have you had morning sickness?____no____

Describe problems that have affected your food intake. nausea

Number of previous pregnancies none

End of last pregnancy NA

Weight gained during last completed pregnancy NA

Describe any complications during previous pregnancies. NO

Do you plan to breast-feed or bottle-feed your baby? breastfeed

Have you breast-fed before? no

If yes, for how long?

Explain why you stopped breastfeeding.

Describe your eating patterns, the meals and snacks you eat and when you eat them. Any time whenever I feel hungry.

Do you frequently eat away from home? no.

List where and what kinds of foods. fruits, cereals, milk, rice, wheat products etc.

List common foods and beverages you do *not* eat, such as milk or meat.

meat, diary products

List ten foods you eat several times a week. fruits, Rice, gram, wheat products, vegetables, milk, cereal, cookies, dry fruits, shakes.

Are you on any special diet, e.g., weight loss, diabetic, vegetarian? no

If yes, describe the type of diet.

Do you drink caffeine-containing beverages (coffee, tea, cola, etc.)? no

If yes, how many per day? —

Do you drink alcoholic beverages? —

If yes, how much? —

How often? —

Do you smoke cigarettes? —

If yes, how many per day? —

Do you use any "recreational" drugs? —

Describe types of exercise you do. walking, streching Aerobics etc

How often? every day

Time spent per exercise session? 1/2 hr.

AGE

Biologically speaking, a "mature woman" is eighteen to thirty-five years old—prime time for meeting the physical challenges of pregnancy. The age range of twenty-five to thirty-four is statistically the most successful time for pregnancy (202). Nevertheless, one out of every four first-time mothers in the United States is under twenty years old, and one out of every four is above age thirty. It isn't unusual these days for women in their forties to bear children. Good nutritional management can help minimize problems at all ages.

The Woman under Eighteen

Babies born to teenage mothers tend to weigh less at birth than babies born to older women. The risks increase for women under age fifteen (35).

Younger women have smaller babies who are more likely to be born with health problems because adolescence is a time of significant, nutrient-draining growth, and the additional needs of pregnancy impose nutritional demands that are hard to meet. The mother who is still growing herself competes with her baby for body-building raw materials. Too often, both end up getting less than what they need. Low-birth-weight babies (those weighing less than five and a half pounds) are more likely to have mental and physical handicaps. Some of these babies never catch up as they mature and require a great deal of special care.

Young women who follow the prevalent diet of teens—who eat infrequent or irregular meals that are heavy on fries and soft drinks and light on fresh fruits, vegetables, and milk—deprive their babies of nourishment. The risks increase if a pregnant teen smokes, drinks alcohol, or experiments with drugs.

Young mothers *can* produce healthy, normal-birth-weight babies, but it takes special effort. If you are under age eighteen and are pregnant, you need to eat enough food to provide for both your own and your baby's growth. Because your baby grows twenty-four hours a day, you have to think about eating at regular times. If you skip meals or diet, you deprive your baby of the nutrients it needs.

The Montreal Diet Dispensary has had good results working with young pregnant women. Participants in their model program are given milk, eggs, oranges, and a vitamin-mineral supplement. No other changes in eating habits are required, yet the chances of having normal-weight babies are better than the average for mothers in this age group (89). The specific food additions provided added protein, B_{12}, calcium, and vitamin C—nutrients that are likely to be in short supply during pregnancy. They also boost calories and vitamin-mineral levels, thus supporting a better nutrient supply to both the baby and the young mother.

Often, teenagers don't think much about what they eat. But when you are having a baby, what you eat makes a big difference!

The Woman over Thirty-five

Years ago it was rare for a woman to have a child after age forty. But now that the average life expectancy of American women has almost doubled, many women spend their early adult years devoting time to getting an education, pursuing a career, and building a relationship with a caring partner. By the time they decide to start a family, these women usually are highly motivated to do everything possible to ensure a successful pregnancy.

While it often takes women over 35 longer to conceive (four to six months is the average), statistically they are no more likely to deliver preterm or low-birth-weight babies. In fact, women in their thirties have fewer low-birth-weight babies than do younger women (116). And older women are less likely than those under age twenty to have anemia, premature labor, and complications during delivery (14).

The results of a study of almost four thousand women showed that, as a whole, having a child after age thirty-five is more of a risk to the mother than the baby (14). Older women who are having a first baby are more likely than younger women to experience bleeding during pregnancy and complications that warrant cesarean delivery, such as abrupt detachment of the placenta or placenta previa (the placenta located so that it covers the opening of the uterus) (14). But age alone does not warrant cesarean delivery. A woman should choose a physician who will cooperate with her to the fullest extent before making a surgical delivery.

Some of the risks of older childbearing have more to do with disease and chronic disorders associated with mid-life, such as hypertension and diabetes, than with the reproductive process itself (14). General health screening should be a part of a prepregnancy checkup for women over age thirty. Potential medical problems can then be monitored and controlled.

The risks of Down's syndrome and other birth defects do increase very gradually with age, but there is no sudden sharp increase, as was formerly thought. More than 97 percent of women who have prenatal diagnostic tests find that their fetus is free from this defect (116). Women are routinely given diagnostic tests that can identify chromosomal damage and detect some potential birth defects. Chromosomal abnormalities play an important role in miscarriages, which do occur more frequently in older women. Prenatal testing also can identify multiple births. The chance for having twins or triplets increases with age, peaking at age thirty-seven.

RACIAL AND ETHNIC ORIGIN

African-American women tend to gain less weight during pregnancy, and to have smaller babies than Caucasian women even when mothers gain the same amount of weight (172). The reason for this difference is unknown (172). Thus, the target weight gain for African-American mothers is set at the high end of the recommended range, unless the mother is very overweight at conception (172).

Ethnic groups with small average body size also have lower weight gains. As succeeding generations grow taller, their babies are born heavier, thus bearing out the relationship between mother's height and weight and baby's birth weight. Statistically, very few low-birth-weight babies are born to Hispanic women (202).

Interestingly, Chinese and Filipino women born outside the United States experience better pregnancies than women of these ethnic origins who are born in the United States. Chinese mothers with low, rather than high, educational levels have been found to have better pregnancies. Stella Wu, a researcher at Hood College in Maryland, attributes this statistic to the lower incidence of risk factors (smoking, alcohol, etc.) among less educated and more recently emigrated women (203).

Many African-American, Hispanic, Native American, and

Asian women are lactose intolerant, which limits their intake of calcium and vitamin D from food. If you do not drink milk, a registered dietitian or your doctor can help you plan alternative ways to get the calcium and vitamin D you need when you are pregnant. In addition, there is evidence that women of color synthesize vitamin D from sunlight more slowly than light-skinned women do (172). Women of *all* races and ethnic groups who are not routinely exposed to sunlight need to consider dietary sources of this important vitamin. Vitamins are discussed more in chapter 5.

PREVIOUS PREGNANCIES

First pregnancies tend to have more complications than later ones (202). The risks increase with five or more pregnancies, especially if they are spaced closely together. Closely spaced pregnancies deplete a woman's iron, folate, and calcium stores, jeopardizing both mother and baby. It takes several months for your body to recover after pregnancy and be in optimal condition to bear another child. If you are breast-feeding, or have recently finished breast-feeding, nutrient stores may be depleted.

If you gained an abnormal amount of weight during your previous pregnancies, or your baby's birth weight and condition required special care, you may be susceptible to nutrition-related problems. For instance, if your babies have been unusually heavy at birth, your doctor will be concerned about gestational diabetes. If previous babies were very small, you may be advised to gain more weight in future pregnancies.

PREVIOUS NUTRITIONAL STATUS

You Are What Your Mother Ate

If you are short (five feet one inch or less) or thin, it may be because you come from a family in which this frame is a genetic trait. But after genetics, the primary determinant of growth is the nutritional adequacy of food you eat during the early growing years and your mother's habits during her pregnancy. If a mother is poorly nourished or smokes during pregnancy, her children may be smaller at birth than genetics would predict. These children have to catch up during the growing years to reach their genetic potential. Animal studies show that poor nutrition stunts growth and that it may take two or three generations before the size of the mother returns to normal and her female offspring give birth to normal-weight babies (197). You will want to do everything you can when you are pregnant so that you don't perpetuate a cycle created by poor nutrition.

You Are What You Ate

Before you blame your mother for your physical imperfections, take a good look at your own eating habits. It may be that, as you were growing up, you always skipped breakfast or ate a candy bar instead of a sandwich at lunch, in spite of your mother's persistent urgings.

An inadequate amount of food, too little calcium, or erratic dieting during your prime growing period may have prevented your bones from growing to their maximum size. Are you or have you ever been anorexic or bulimic? Do you have a history of dieting—avoiding milk or not eating meat because you thought they were fattening? Did you refuse to eat anything that didn't come in a box or a bag? Seemingly innocuous eating practices make a difference to the resources you bring to pregnancy.

Weight and Height

Weight-for-height at the time of conception is a better indicator of maternal nutritional status than weight alone (172). Both your height and weight will be measured at your prepregnancy checkup or first prenatal visit. Height should be measured early in pregnancy, before your body posture changes, using a stadiometer, which is more accurate than the measuring instrument on a scale.

Maternal height correlates directly with birth weight, regardless of the amount of weight the mother gains during pregnancy (197). Women who are shorter than five feet two inches gain on average two pounds less than women who are taller than five feet seven inches, but there is no evidence that short women are at greater risk of inadequate weight gain.

Weight should be measured by someone trained in the proper procedure, using a platform beam balance scale with movable weights or a calibrated electronic scale. Your weight will be measured each time you see your doctor. Sometimes the procedure is to weigh patients in paper examining gowns; sometimes patients are weighed wearing light, indoor clothing. (Some of us routinely slip off wristwatch, earrings, and belt before stepping on a scale.) For consistency, wear the same type of clothing each time you are weighed. It's hard to set a realistic target weight gain without accurate prepregnancy measurements.

Your doctor may use a complex chart based on body mass

index (BMI) to determine whether you are underweight, normal, or overweight. The weight-for-height table on pages 10–11 can be used as a general guide. It's important to take actual measurements, though, because studies show (172) that women tend to underestimate their weight and overestimate their height!

As discussed in the last chapter, your doctor will record your prepregnant weight and chart subsequent gains at each prenatal visit.

TWINS, TRIPLETS, ETC.

If you are having twins or triplets, your doctor will monitor your pregnancy closely and help you determine appropriate adjustments to your diet. Though the actual quantity of needed nutrients is not yet known, the general information about nutrients in this book still applies. You can assume that your babies demand more of virtually all nutrients. A high-quality diet, perhaps with a balanced prenatal supplement, will protect you and your infants.

There are specific concerns related to twin pregnancies (172).

- Mothers of twins tend to gain too little weight, especially if they do not know until late in their pregnancy that they are carrying more than one baby.
- Many twins have low birth weights, even when carried to term.
- Nonidentical twins are more likely to weigh different amounts than are identical twins.
- Many twins are born preterm—usually two to three weeks early.

- Women who carry twins are more likely to experience certain complications (anemia, pregnancy-induced hypertension).
- Cesarean delivery is more common in twin births.

Twins are limited in size by the total blood supply to the placenta and the degree to which the uterus can expand, as well as by the mother's age, prepregnancy condition, and genetic make-up. Birth weight is generally lower in female infants, in first pregnancies, and in infants born to women who smoke (172). On average, a mother carrying twins gains four to nine pounds more than the mother of a single baby (172). A 1989 study done in Seattle reported that the average weight gain for mothers who bore healthy, full-term twins was forty-four pounds. Mothers who gained less had poorer outcomes and smaller babies.

EATING HABITS

Skipping breakfast, having a quick snack at your desk, and eating a burger and fries in the car may be your practice, but it is not good for baby-building. During every single minute of your pregnancy, from conception until birth, cells are dividing and growing. Your baby needs a ready supply of energy and high-quality nutrients to develop into a healthy human being. Pregnancy is a time for eating regularly, eating well, and eating often. Chapter 3 presents an eating "game plan."

If you have diabetes, high blood pressure, or other medical problems, or must restrict food choices for other reasons, you will need special prenatal guidance to meet both your medical and nutritional needs. Talk with a registered dietitian who can help you make adjustments for pregnancy.

EXERCISE

Physical conditioning is as important to good health during pregnancy as it is when you are not pregnant. There are many benefits to exercise: It maintains muscle tone, strength, and endurance; protects against back pain; and promises a positive effect on energy level, mood, and self-image. An exercise program that is approved and monitored by your doctor can help promote fitness during pregnancy. The more active you are, the more calories you can eat without gaining excessive weight.

Many contemporary women have made vigorous exercise a part of their lives and want to continue a high level of activity throughout pregnancy. Our friend Nancy, a triathalon athlete, "geared down" during pregnancy to a twenty-five-mile-a-day bike ride—a regimen she continued right up to delivery. While Nancy and her baby are both strong and healthy, experts usually advise women to decrease the duration, frequency, and/or intensity of vigorous exercise, especially during the last trimester (202).

The American College of Obstetricians and Gynecologists (ACOG) provides specific guidelines for exercise during pregnancy (3). Based on the unique physical and physiological conditions of pregnancy and the postpartum period, they help pregnant women develop safe home exercise programs. We reprint them with permission of the ACOG and suggest that you discuss them with your doctor.

PREGNANCY AND POSTPARTUM EXERCISE

1. Regular exercise (at least three times per week) is preferable to intermittent activity. Competitive activities should be discouraged.

2. Vigorous exercise should not be performed in hot, humid weather or during a period of febrile illness [when you have a fever].

3. Ballistic movements (jerky, bouncy motions) should be avoided. Exercise should be done on a wooden floor or a tightly carpeted surface to reduce shock and provide a sure footing.

4. Deep flexion or extension of joints should be avoided because of connective tissue laxity. [Connective tissues are more elastic during pregnancy.] Activities that require jumping, jarring motions, or rapid changes in direction should be avoided because of joint instability.

5. Vigorous exercise should be preceded by a five-minute period of muscle warm-up. This can be accomplished by slow walking or stationary cycling with low resistance.

6. Vigorous exercise should be followed by a period of gradually declining activity that includes gentle stationary stretching. Because connective tissue laxity increases the risk of joint injury, stretches should not be taken to the point of maximum resistance.

7. Heart rate should be measured at times of peak activity. Target heart rates and limits established in consultation with the physician should not be exceeded.

8. Maternal core temperature should not exceed 38°C (99°F).

This is not the time for a no pain–no gain philosophy of exercise. You should discuss all exercise-related questions with your doctor. If you have any of the following symptoms, stop exercising and contact your doctor.

Pain
Faintness
Bleeding
Tachycardia [abnormal, rapid heartbeat]
Dizziness
Back pain
Shortness of breath
Pubic pain [or any cramping]
Palpitations
Difficulty walking

The last months of pregnancy put a great strain on your circulatory system. If you do strenuous physical exercise or work, your muscles will compete with the placenta for blood. This can strain your heart and increase the risk of premature delivery. Your doctor will help you to determine an appropriate program of physical activity for pregnancy.

Physical activity can improve your appetite, reduce stress, and help you sleep better. A brisk walk, perhaps with some portable music, is one of the best ways to exercise during pregnancy. There are a number of excellent books and videos on exercise during pregnancy, and a variety of classes are available in most communities. Healthy pregnant women have come out of the closet and are dancing, stretching, running, skiing, biking, and walking to the delivery room.

3

An Eating Game Plan

QUICK QUIZ

STEP 1

Write down on a piece of paper every food that you ate or drank yesterday from the time you woke up until you went to sleep. Be sure to include snacks and beverages, even water.

STEP 2

Look at each of the foods you listed. On the table below, make one mark in the "Your Intake" column for each serving of any item you ate yesterday. Give one mark for a regular-sized portion; for example, a side-dish size salad would get only one mark even if it contained three ingredients—lettuce, tomatoes, and cucumber; two cups of coffee with breakfast would get two marks even though you drank both at the same meal; a sandwich would get two bread marks plus marks for the filling; pasta as a main course gets 2–3 marks. Add the marks you made in each group and write it on the "Total for day" line to find how many servings you had in each of the six groups.

	FOODS	YOUR INTAKE
GROUP 1:	Milk (also credit GROUP 6)	
	Yogurt	
	Cheese	
	Ice cream	

	FOODS	YOUR INTAKE
	Puddings, custard	
	Other dairy products	
	Total for day	______
GROUP 2:	Fresh fruit	
	Fruit juice (also credit GROUP 6)	
	Canned fruit	
	Raw vegetable or salad	
	Dried fruit	
	Other fruits or vegetables	
	Total for day	______
GROUP 3:	Bread, roll, bagel, etc.	
	Cereal	
	Grain, rice	
	Noodles, pasta	
	Total for day	______
GROUP 4:	Meat	
	Fish or poultry	
	Dried beans or peas	
	Nuts	
	Eggs	
	Other protein foods	
	Total for day	______
GROUP 5:	Sugar	
	Sweets, candy	
	Salad dressing	

	FOODS	YOUR INTAKE
	Butter or margarine	
	Cream	
	Fried food (also credit the food type: e.g., fried chicken, also credit Group 4)	
	Total for day	______
Group 6:	Water, 1 glass	
	Milk (also credit Group 1)	
	Fruit juice (also credit Group 2)	
	Coffee or tea	
	Soft drinks	
	Other beverages	
	Total for day	______

How many glasses of beer, wine, spirits, or other beverages containing alcohol did you have yesterday?______ Do you drink more on weekends?______

List foods that do not fit any of the above groups.____________

____

____

____

____

____

STEP 3

Sit down, put your feet up, and read this chapter.

STEP 4
Now evaluate yesterday's food intake on the basis of what you need. How close were you to the recommended number of servings for each group listed on page 50. Are there whole groups of foods you do not eat? What two changes can you make to improve your diet tomorrow?

In this chapter, we are going to move our discussion to the supermarket, the cafeteria, the restaurant, the kitchen, the dinner party—places where you make food choices.

Years of experience in dietary counseling have convinced us that diet plans must be individualized. There are diets that call for specific foods on a schedule. Many of them are very nutritious—on paper. But if the foods listed never make it to your mouth, the diet is not nutritious for you or your baby. What good is it to tell you to eat something you do not like, do not know how to prepare, or cannot afford to buy?

With an eating game plan, you can assess your strengths and weaknesses, so you can make substitutions where necessary. Guided by this book, you can work at making good food choices every day. Feeling good during and after pregnancy and having a healthy baby make it well worth the effort.

A DIET THAT WORKS

A diet that works

- Is based on your habits, preferences, and needs
- Provides information so that you can make rational food choices based on fact

- Gives you a gentle push in the right direction by telling you about the benefits of good eating and warning you about potential dangers

Ethnic background, income, ease of preparation, cooking skills and equipment, food preferences of other family members, frequency of meals away from home, and taste preferences are just some of the factors that influence your food choices. Pregnancy brings a new awareness to these choices.

It's not just a myth that pregnant women get cravings for specific tastes. There may be a physiological reason for a craving. Women who crave nonfood substances such as cornstarch or ice may have an iron deficiency (see page 176). There is evidence that salt cravings may also be physiologic in nature; hence the desire for pickles.

Foods that pregnant women crave may bring comfort and joy—pretty essential "nutrients" in our thinking! Mary had cravings for Gorgonzola cheese and figs in the evening, during one pregnancy, and discovered several years later, while traveling in Italy, that this is a classic Italian combination.

A diet that works balances good nutrition with personal preferences and considers your emotional as well as physical needs.

Hey, Dad! You're Eating for Two, Too

Having a baby is a family affair. One of the most significant ways a father can become involved is to take an active and supportive role in the mother's prenatal diet. There's a lot to learn about all the nutrients and their roles in pregnancy. Prospective parents can read this book together and discuss its implications for their meal planning. If dietary changes are necessary, it will be easier to make them together. *Pregnancy is a good time to improve the eating patterns of the entire family.* With few exceptions, what is good for mother and baby during pregnancy will be good for everyone in the family. It may be wise for other family members to limit foods rich in cholesterol and saturated fat and to reduce their intake of salt.

The father can be helpful in these ways:

- Encourage regular eating patterns. This effort may mean that you will end up being responsible for preparing or bringing home some of the meals.
- Play milkman. Make sure there's a quart a day (or its equivalent) exclusively for Mom.
- Remind Mom to take her prenatal supplement, if one is prescribed.
- Bring home beautiful fresh fruits and vegetables along with an occasional bouquet of flowers.
- Help shop for nutritious foods. Be willing to try new foods.
- If morning sickness strikes, remember you are partially responsible! Do what you can by providing moral support and crackers, with love and understanding. Do not expect her to make your breakfast! Make breakfast for other family members.
- When eating out, encourage Mom to order foods that are good for her which might not be prepared at home. How about a chopped liver appetizer or calves' liver and onions?
- Don't fill the house with food you want to eat but Mom wants to avoid.

THE BEST CHOICES IN THE SIX FOOD GROUPS

To help you select foods that will provide the nutrients you need, we have divided foods into groups and have suggested the number of selections from each group that make up a balanced diet. *A balanced diet is one that provides all of the essential nutrients within a reasonable calorie limit from a variety of foods.*

In recent years, agencies of the federal government have promoted a food guide that splits fruits and vegetables into separate groups. Because the nutrients from fruits and vegetables are similar, we have kept them as one group to simplify our advice to you.

In school, you may have learned about the *four* basic food groups. We have expanded our list to *six* food groups. The added groups help you to meet your need for water and other liquids and to choose fats and sugars that make your food tasty and enjoyable. The food groups are

1. Milk and dairy products
2. Fruits and vegetables
3. Breads and cereals
4. Protein foods
5. Fats and sugars
6. Water and other liquids

Your needs during pregnancy are different from those of children or adult men. The Daily Food Guide chart is adapted from the Daily Food Guide promoted by the federal government as part of "Dietary Guidelines for Americans," which has been endorsed by the American Dietetic Association (1).

The chart below shows the recommended number of servings for you and other members of your family. A plus sign (+) means "or more."

DAILY FOOD GUIDE

	PREGNANT WOMEN	NON-PREGNANT WOMEN	MEN	CHILDREN
1. Milk and dairy products	4+	2+	2+	2–3+
2. Fruits and vegetables vitamin C-rich	1+	1	1	1
deep green, yellow, or orange	2	3+ per wk	3+ per wk	3+ per wk
other	3+	2+	2+	2+
Daily total	6+	5+	5+	5+
3. Breads and cereals	6+	6+	6+	6+
4. Protein foods	3	2	2	2
5. Fats and sugars	As necessary for added calories			
6. Water, other liquids	8+	6–8	6–8	6–8

In the following pages, we list Best Choices and Other Choices in each food group based on the density of nutrients in the food. We calculated nutrient density by giving pluses for the positive nutritional content in a food, and minuses for added sugar, salt, cholesterol, or saturated fat. Nutrient-dense foods have far more pluses than minuses.

Best Choices provide lots of nutrients without significant calories from added sugar or fat. If you are having a problem controlling your weight, make almost all of your food choices from this group. *Other Choices* contribute to recommended servings from a food group, but they have either smaller amounts of key nutrients or added sugar and fat.

Food Group 1: Milk and Dairy Products

Four or more servings are needed each day. Women carrying twins should have six or more servings daily (1).

One serving equals

1 cup of milk
1 cup of yogurt
1½ oz. hard cheese, such as Cheddar or Swiss
1 cup soft cheese, such as cottage or ricotta
½ cup ice cream, pudding, custard
1 cup frozen yogurt

Some of the foods you might expect to find listed here are not. Butter, cream, sour cream, and coffee lighteners all have lots of fat but are low in calcium, phosphorus, protein, riboflavin, and other nutrients provided by this group; therefore, they don't count as milk servings but as fats.

Ice cream can be a part of a nutritious diet, but keep in mind that it takes two cups of regular vanilla ice cream, with a whopping 538 calories (or 698 calories of super-rich vanilla ice cream), to get the same amount of calcium as is in a glass of skim milk, which contains only 86 calories!

Although we look to milk to meet calcium needs, milk also provides an inexpensive source of complete protein. Instant nonfat dry milk (powdered skim milk) is a particularly economical source of many nutrients. If you mix it and refrigerate it for a few hours, the flavor is better. Mix about a cup of whole milk into a quart of reconstituted dry milk for do-it-yourself 1 percent lowfat milk.

Milk and Dairy Products

Best Choices

Buttermilk
Cottage, pot, farmer, or ricotta cheese
Evaporated whole or skim milk
Lactaid® (if lactose-intolerant)
Lowfat frozen yogurt
Lowfat kefir
Lowfat (1% or 2%) milk
Lowfat or nonfat yogurt
Nonfat dry milk
Part-skim cheeses (e.g., mozzarella)
Reduced-fat cheeses
Skim milk

Other Choices*

Cheesecake
Cheeses (e.g., Cheddar, Swiss, Muenster)
Chocolate milk
Creamed soups
Custard
Eggnog (pasteurized)
Flavored yogurt
Frozen yogurt (regular)
Ice cream
Ice milk
Milkshake

OTHER CHOICES* *continued*

Pudding	Whole milk
Quiche	Whole-milk yogurt

* Some foods on this list—ice cream, for instance—are also on lists of foods high in sugar and/or fat.

In the last few years, calcium-fortified juices (orange, grapefruit and apple juice) have become available. If you are intolerant of or do not eat dairy products, consider these juices. But remember, they have the calcium but not the protein, vitamins, and minerals present in dairy products. Another way to boost calcium is to choose calcium-fortified milk that doubles the calcium level per glass. Evaporated milk (both whole and skim) is on our Best Choice list because it contains twice as much calcium and other nutrients per ounce as regular milk. It is a good substitute for cream.

Reduced-fat cheeses clearly belong on the Best Choice list, as do low-fat cheeses now found in supermarkets. Soft cheeses and all forms of cottage cheese, even creamed cottage cheese, are in this category. If you don't particularly enjoy milk, boost calcium by putting feta or parmesan cheese in salads and part-skim mozzarella on sandwiches. Cheeses like Lorraine Swiss and Jarlsberg are moderate in fat. Many brand name natural and processed reduced-fat cheeses are available that have only five grams of fat per ounce. Most provide nutrient information on the label and are good choices. Most hard cheeses, however, like Cheddar, American, and Gouda, are quite high in fat, but they do provide lots of important minerals and vitamins. Very rich cheeses such as cream cheese are primarily fat and appear in food group 5 with other fats. Our advice is to avoid too much fat by choosing lowfat meats and skim milk on days you have full-fat cheeses. If you are having trouble gaining enough weight, consider hard cheeses a Best Choice for getting some extra calories.

CHEESE COMPARISONS (PER 1 OZ. PORTION)

	GRAMS FAT	MILLIGRAMS CALCIUM	CALORIES
American (processed)	8.9	124	106
Blue	8.2	150	100
Brick	8.4	191	105
Brie	7.9	52	95
Camembert	6.9	110	85
Cheddar	9.4	204	114
Colby	9.1	194	112
Cottage cheese			
creamed	1.3	17	29
lowfat, 2% fat	0.6	19	25
dry curd	0.1	10	24
Cream cheese	9.9	20	99
Edam	7.9	207	101
Feta	6.0	140	75
Gouda	7.8	198	101
Gruyère	9.2	287	117
Havarti	10.6	176	121
Limburger	7.7	141	93
Monterey Jack	8.6	212	106
Mozzarella (part skim)	4.5	183	72
Muenster	8.5	203	104

	GRAMS FAT	MILLIGRAMS CALCIUM	CALORIES
Neufchâtel	6.6	21	74
Parmesan	7.3	336	111
Provolone	7.6	214	100
Ricotta			
part skim	2.2	75	39
whole milk	3.6	56	49
Romano	7.6	302	110
Roquefort	8.7	188	105
String or Strip cheese	5.0	200	80
Swiss	7.8	272	107
Swiss (processed)	7.1	219	95

Food Group 2: Fruits and Vegetables

Choose six or more servings of fruits and vegetables each day. At least two of these servings should be fresh fruit or raw vegetables.

One serving equals

½ cup raw fruit or vegetable
1 cup green salad or raw leafy greens
½ cup canned fruit
½ cup cooked fruit or vegetable
6 oz. juice
1 medium-sized piece of fruit or vegetable

Both fruits and vegetables supply important vitamins, including A, C, and folate, as well as minerals and fiber. Because this food group must supply several key nutrients, there are Best Choices listed for both vitamins A and C. Try to choose a Best Choice Vitamin C fruit or vegetable each day, and do the same for Vitamin A-rich fruits and vegetables.

Some fruits and vegetables—cantaloupe and broccoli, for example—appear in both Best Choice columns because they are rich in several nutrients. If you eat one of these foods, you get a nutritional double whammy, but you still need a *total* of at least six servings of fruits and vegetables.

Second Best Choices are foods that are not as high in vitamins A and C as the foods in the Best Choices lists, but they do contribute to the total vitamins, minerals, and fiber that you need each day, and they provide variety and interest. And they don't have added fat or sugar.

The *Other Choices* are fruit and vegetables prepared with fat or sugar. Limit your selections from this group (unless you need to gain weight), and try to balance their higher calorie content by making other prudent food choices during the day.

Fruits

Best Choices

VITAMIN C

Acerola cherry
Cantaloupe
Cranberry juice (fortified)
Grapefruit
Guava
Kiwi
Lemon
Mango
Orange
Orange juice
Papaya
Strawberries
Tangerine
Tangerine juice

Best Choices (continued)

VITAMIN A (DEEP GREEN, YELLOW, OR ORANGE)

Apricot
Cantaloupe
Mango
Papaya
Pumpkin

Second-Best Choices

Apple
Apple juice or cider
Applesauce (unsweetened)
Avocado
Banana
Blackberries
Blueberries
Boysenberries
Casaba melon
Cherries
Currants
Dates
Dried fruit
Figs
Grape juice
Grapes
Honeydew melon
Nectarine
Peach
Pear
Persimmon
Pineapple
Pineapple juice
Plantain
Plum
Prune juice
Prunes
Raisins
Raspberries
Rhubarb
Watermelon

Other Choices

Applesauce (sweetened)
Canned fruits, especially those canned in heavy syrup
Fruit drinks (orange drink, etc.)
Fruit nectars (apricot, pear, etc.)
Fruit pies, cobblers, or crisps
Lemonade

Vegetables

Best Choices

VITAMIN C

Broccoli
Brussels sprouts
Cabbage, green or red
Cauliflower
Green pepper
Kale
Rutabaga
Spinach
Sweet potato
Swiss chard
Tomato

VITAMIN A (DEEP GREEN, YELLOW, OR ORANGE)

Beet greens
Broccoli
Brussels sprouts
Carrot
Chicory
Collard greens
Dandelion greens
Escarole
Kale
Lettuces (dark-green)
Mixed vegetables
Mustard greens
Spinach
Sweet potato
Swiss chard
Winter squash (acorn, hubbard, butternut)

Second-Best Choices

Alfalfa sprouts
Artichoke
Asparagus
Beans (kidney, garbanzo, green beans, limas, wax beans, bean sprouts)
Beets
Celery
Corn
Cucumber
Eggplant
Kohlrabi
Leeks

Second Best-Choices (continued)

Lettuce (iceberg)
Mushrooms
Okra
Parsnip
Peas
Potato
Radishes
Scallions
Summer squash
Turnips
Yams

Other Choices

Deep-fried vegetables
Potato chips, potato sticks, potato salad
Salads with excessive dressing
Sauerkraut
Vegetables frozen in sauces
Vegetables in cream sauce

Food Group 3: Breads and Cereals

Choose six or more servings from this group each day.

One serving equals

1 slice bread
1 muffin or tortilla
½ English muffin, bun or bagel
1 small roll or biscuit
½ cup cooked cereal
¾–1 cup (1 oz.) ready-to-eat cereal
½ cup rice, noodles, spaghetti, grits
4–8 crackers, depending on size

Breads and cereals are made from grains. Some grain products are made from the whole kernel of the grain. Most, however, are more highly processed and use only part of the grain kernel.

Whole-grain products made from the whole kernel, such as rye and whole-wheat flour, are the most nutritious. In milling and processing, fiber, folate, pantothenic acid, vitamin E, B vitamins, magnesium, manganese, iron, copper, potassium, and chromium are removed. Whole grains retain these nutrients.

Highly processed flour is used in most breads and cereals. In milling wheat, the *bran,* which is the outer covering of the kernel, and the *germ,* the innermost part, are removed. The result is *white flour.* Vitamins, minerals, and dietary fiber are lost when the bran and germ are removed. Flour and other foods can be treated to add nutrients; they can be *fortified* or *enriched.* The label will tell you if either has been done.

Enriched

In processing the grain, much of the fiber, many vitamins, and minerals are removed. Enrichment returns only three vitamins—thiamin, riboflavin, and niacin—and one mineral—iron—to enriched products. Actual enrichment levels are determined by food laws. Most flour and many breads are enriched.

Fortified

In fortification, vitamins, minerals, and sometimes protein that were not in the original food are added as the food is processed. Many breakfast cereals are fortified.

If you regularly eat a fortified cereal in addition to taking a prenatal multivitamin, be sure to tell your doctor. Some fortified cereals contain as much as 100 percent of the U.S. RDA for specific nutrients, so it may be desirable to omit the balanced prenatal supplement and take only iron to avoid oversupplementation.

The Best Choices list for breads and cereals is divided into whole-grain and enriched or fortified foods. Although whole-grain bread has many advantages, it also contains phytic acid, which can reduce the absorption of several minerals. Nevertheless, the benefits far outweigh this disadvantage, and whole-grain bread should be included in your diet every day.

Breads and Cereals

Best Choices

WHOLE GRAIN

Barley
Brown rice
Corn tortilla (not fried)
Millet
Mixed-grain and whole-wheat crackers
Multi-grain bread
Popcorn, unbuttered
Pumpernickel bread†
Rye bread or crackers†
Wheat germ
Whole-grain cereals, hot or cold (oatmeal, shredded wheat, etc.)
Whole-grain waffles
Whole-wheat bread, rolls, pita
Whole-wheat pastas
Wild rice

ENRICHED/FORTIFIED

Bagel
Bialy roll
Biscuits
Bread, rolls, buns, pita
Bread sticks
Cereals (without excessive sugar)
Cornbread, corn muffins‡

ENRICHED/FORTIFIED

Corn grits	Mixed-grain cereals
English muffins	Pancakes, waffles
Farina	Pasta, macaroni, noodles
Flour tortilla	Puffed wheat or rice
Graham crackers	White rice

OTHER CHOICES

Biscuits	Granola
Bread or rice pudding	Highly sugared cereals (more than 8 grams of sugar per serving)
Bread stuffing	Macaroni, pasta salads
Cookies	Muffins
Croissants	Tortilla chips
Doughnuts, sweet rolls	White breads (not labeled enriched)
French and Italian breads (not labeled enriched)	
Fruit breads, nut breads	

* Items on this list assume "typical" preparation. Some can be prepared with whole-grain or enriched flour, low-fat contents, and reduced sugar to improve their nutritional profile.

† Rye bread or crackers and pumpernickel *may* be made with whole grain, but many are made primarily with enriched white flour and have added coloring.

‡ Corn bread and muffins, if made from stone-ground corn meal are whole grain, but may have large amounts of fat and sugar.

Food Group 4: Protein Foods

It's best to have a good source of complete protein at each meal—or three servings of high-quality protein food, besides milk, each day.

One serving* equals

3 oz. cooked lean meat, poultry, or fish
2 eggs
1 cup cooked dry peas, beans, soybeans, or lentils
4 tbsp. peanut butter
$\frac{1}{3}$ cup nuts, sesame seeds, or sunflower seeds
8 oz. tofu (soybean curd)

* All foods on this list provide some high-quality protein. The amount of protein varies. So does the amount of fat. It is wise to include a variety of foods from the protein food lists, thus balancing high- and low-fat and low-cholesterol choices within the group. Refer to the protein chart in chapter 4 for equivalent amounts.

Protein Foods

Best Choices

ANIMAL

Chicken
Cornish game hen
Eggs and egg substitutes
Fish
Lean beef, lamb, pork, veal
Liver, organ meats
Liver sausage
Shellfish (shrimp, oysters, lobster, crab)
Turkey, turkey ham

VEGETABLE

Black-eyed peas
Garbanzo beans
Kidney beans
Lentils
Lima beans
Pea beans
Pinto beans
Split peas

Best Choices (continued)

VEGETABLE

Soybeans
Textured vegetable protein (TVP)
Tofu (soybean curd)

Other Choices

ANIMAL

Bologna
Cold cuts
Corned beef
Duck
Fish sticks, breaded
Fried chicken
Fried fish
Fried meats
Goose
Hamburger (not lean)
Salami
Sausages, frankfurters
Shortribs and fatty cuts of beef
Spareribs and other fatty cuts of pork

VEGETABLE

Almond butter
Nuts
Peanut butter
Sesame seeds
Sunflower seeds

The American Heart Association and the Dietary Guidelines for Americans suggest that it would be prudent for the general population to limit consumption of eggs and other sources of cholesterol, but we encourage you to eat eggs because they are a quick, easy, economical source of protein and other key nutrients, and cholesterol is not a major concern for most women during pregnancy (see chapter 4). You may want to eat more eggs than do other family members.

A vegetarian who eats no meat, poultry, or fish but consumes a wide range of grains, legumes, nuts, fruits, vegetables, and dairy products can have a nutritionally adequate diet for her own and her baby's needs. For vegetarians, one egg, one cup of legumes or tofu, and four glasses of milk (or the equivalent in cheese) each day go a long way in meeting protein needs during pregnancy. The remaining protein needs can be met with grains, nuts, seeds, and vegetables.

Vegetarians who do not eat eggs or use other dairy products have a more difficult time getting adequate protein, iron, zinc, calcium, and vitamin B_{12}. If enough grains and vegetables are chosen, protein needs can be met, although supplementary vitamins and minerals may be required. Since iron absorption is boosted by vitamin C eaten at the same meal, it is wise to eat a fruit or vegetable at every meal to maximize iron usage. Nutrition evaluation and a consulting session with a registered dietitian may be particularly beneficial for vegetarians. Again, we emphasize that *it is important for the vegetarian mother-to-be to consume adequate calories so that the protein she eats will not be used to meet energy needs* (see chapter 4).

Food Group 5: Fats and Oils, Sugars and Sweets

Most nutrition-conscious women strive to limit the fat and sugar they eat, so it may be a surprise to see this category listed as part of a healthy pregnancy diet. In fact, you need very little oil or sugar each day. But some fats and sugars must be used in preparing foods to make them taste good. As discussed in chapter 1, you do need calories for proper weight gain, and that's where this category can be useful—especially for those who have a hard time gaining enough weight.

The trick here is moderation. A little bit of butter or margarine may help the green beans go down, but very often, the little bit gets to be a lot. One tablespoon of regular salad dressing has seventy to eighty-five calories and nine grams of fat, about the amount of fat in two teaspoons of margarine. Labels currently list one tablespoon as the standard portion, but many people use four tablespoons of dressing, thus adding three hundred calories and a whole day's fat requirement to one salad. Either use as little as possible regular dressing—some people eat it on the side and dip the greens—or substitute a low-calorie or fat-free dressing.

If you choose a low-calorie dressing, you can have far more for the same number of calories (and fat) as the "standard" portion. Low-calorie dressings that use yogurt or buttermilk as a base add extra nutrients while avoiding excess calories.

Because consumers have responded to recommendations to limit fat, food manufacturers have developed many new low-fat products. New fat replacers are coming to the market. In some cases, as with some low-fat, cholesterol-free baked goods, fat has been omitted and the mouth feel of fat is created by special techniques of mixing and the use of edible carbohydrate gums and gels. But a sweet roll is still a sweet roll; even without the high fat, it is essentially flour and sugar. It's OK sometimes, as an "other choice," but certainly not a "best choice." On the other hand, lowfat and nonfat frozen yogurts, salad dressings, and cheeses are found on the Best Choice lists.

FOODS WITH DIFFERENT FAT LEVELS

	PORTION	GRAMS FAT	CALORIES
Potatoes boiled (without skin)	1 med.	.1	116
baked (with skin)	2½″ diam.	.2	220
w/cottage cheese	1 tbsp.	1.5	249
w/sour cream	2 tbsp.	5.2	272
w/butter or margarine	1 tbsp.	12.4	328
French fries, homemade	10 pieces	8.3	158
fast food	3 oz. bag	14.2	274
Toast, whole-wheat	1 slice	1.0	61
w/1 tsp. butter or margarine	1 slice	5.1	97
Chicken roast breast (w/o skin)	½ breast	3.1	142
roast breast (w/skin)	½ breast	7.6	193
fried breast (w/o skin)	½ breast	8.7	218

	PORTION	GRAMS FAT	CALORIES
fried wings (w/skin)	3 wings	21.3	306

The way food is prepared and seasoned can make a big difference in the amount of fat—and calories—you add to your diet. The same is true of sugar. How much sugar do you add to your breakfast cereal? Do you choose an apple (81 calories) or apple pie (282 calories)? We aren't suggesting cutting out apple pie entirely; just use the high-sugar, high-fat alternative less frequently and in a moderate portion.

Look for reduced-fat versions of margarine, salad dressing, mayonnaise, sour cream (sour half-and-half), cream cheese, chips, etc. They have less fat per portion but still count as fats and should be consumed in only moderate amounts. *You do not have to give up your favorite foods—enjoy them in reasonable amounts, and do not overdo on any given day.*

Fats and Oils

Best Choices

Small amounts of:

Butter or margarine, whipped or calorie reduced
Cream cheese, reduced fat
Half and half
Ice cream, regular
Mayonnaise, light or reduced calorie
Salad dressings, reduced calorie
Sour half and half
Vegetable oil, salad oil
Whipped topping

Other Choices

Bagel chips	Ice cream, premium
Butter	Margarine
Cheeses, high fat	Mayonnaise
Corn chips	Potato chips
Cream	Salad dressings
Cream cheese	Sour cream
Fried foods	Tortilla chips
Gravy	

Some of our recommended sweets have nutritionally redeeming ingredients (ice milk, pudding bars). Others are low in fat (angel food cake, ladyfingers). A few teaspoons of sugar, honey, or jam go a long way and have relatively few calories. But who eats two teaspoons of candy or coffee cake? We, too, love pecan pie and brownies, but save them for special occasions, and then in small portions. Even a moderate serving of cake or pie, a sweet roll or rich cheesecake, has several hundred calories and few nutrients. And don't be fooled: Low-fat and fat-free bakery products still have sugar! Some people are surprised to find that flavored gelatin isn't a special health food. It is little more than sugar-sweetened, colored, flavored water.

Sugars and Sweets

Best Choices

Small amounts of:

Angel food cake	Fruited gelatin
Carrot or banana cake	Fruit-flavored yogurt
Fig bars	Gingerbread
Frozen yogurt	Gingersnaps

BEST CHOICES (continued)

Small amounts of:

Graham crackers
Honey
Ice cream
Ice milk
Ladyfingers
Maple syrup
Molasses
Preserves, jam
Pudding bars
Pudding made with lowfat milk
Sugar
Vanilla wafers

OTHER CHOICES

Cakes
Candy
Cookies and brownies
Ice cream
Pies
Regular gelatin
Rich custards

TIPS TO CUT FAT AND SUGAR

- Use one or two tablespoons of dressing on your salad, not a quarter cup. Find a low-calorie or fat-free dressing you like.
- Eat two cookies with your milk instead of six.
- Choose a regular cereal and add one or two teaspoons of sugar if desired instead of eating super-sweetened ready-to-eat cereal.
- Drink real fruit juice instead of sweetened fruit drinks that are just fruit-flavored sugar water.
- Order barbecued instead of fried chicken.
- Use whipped margarine or butter or light margarine as a spread instead of regular margarine or butter.
- Have baked or mashed potatoes instead of French fries.

- On the day you have pie for lunch, eat a piece of fruit for dessert after dinner.
- Choose pudding made with milk and sometimes grain (rice or bread pudding).
- Try a squeeze of lemon on your fish instead of tartar sauce.
- Use mustard or ketchup on sandwiches instead of high-fat "special sauces."

Food Group 6: Water and Other Liquids

The nutrient most vital to human life is a beverage that is usually free, is readily available, requires no preparation, and has no calories—water! Unfortunately, you hear much more about its liquid competitors, which may have won a more prominent place in your diet, than the no-frills product that comes straight from the tap. Few people consciously include water in their diet. You rarely think of it, unless you are deprived of it, yet water is an essential nutrient that must be replenished frequently to sustain life.

More than half of your body—ten to twelve gallons—is water. It assists in absorption, digestion, lubrication, waste removal, and temperature maintenance. Two-and-a-half to three quarts are lost each day, primarily through urination and perspiration. This water must be replaced to keep your system running smoothly. During pregnancy, you need even more water to maintain your expanded blood supply.

Your intake should increase to eight or more glasses each day. If you are not accustomed to drinking water by the glass, this guideline may sound impossible to meet, but there is water in many other liquids you'll be drinking to meet your needs. If you drink four eight-ounce glasses of milk and a glass of juice, you have about five glasses already and need only three more. Some additional liquid comes from solid food. Most fruits and vegetables contain more than 80 percent water, meat and poultry are one-half to two-thirds water, and even bread is one-third water. Liquids such as milk, fruit juice, and soup all help to meet your water needs. Coffee and tea provide water but have a diuretic effect, thus promoting quick loss of water taken in. Most nutrition experts recommend 8–10 cups of water daily.

In many sections of the country, water is the primary source of *fluoride.* Fluoride is the most effective way to prevent tooth decay. Whether or not a pregnant woman's intake of fluoride influences tooth formation is not known, and the relationship of prenatal fluoride to a child's tooth decay is a matter of some dispute (172). Nevertheless, women are encouraged to drink fluoridated water throughout pregnancy (172).

Many women are faced with a real "drinking problem" during pregnancy. If you're not a regular milk drinker, consuming four glasses a day can be a difficult task. Many women limit their water intake to a few sips from a drinking fountain and drink a lot of coffee, tea, or soft drinks. The general rule is to drink one quart of water for every thousand calories of food.

Regular *soft drinks* are loaded with sugar, have many calories and are acidic, contributing to tooth decay. A typical soft drink contains ten teaspoons of sugar! Diet soft drinks don't have sugar or calories but do have considerable amounts of artificial sweeteners, and you may wish to avoid these as well. If you normally drink soft drinks, try to reduce the amount and drink more nutritious beverages instead.

New to the market are flavored seltzers, but they are not

the same as traditional calorie-free carbonated waters. Some flavored seltzers, from kiwi and peach to passion fruit, are sweetened with sugar, corn syrup, or high-fructose syrup and have as many calories as regular soft drinks. Read the label's ingredient panel to see what's in the bottle.

It is quite popular these days to order bottled *mineral water* with fresh lime or lemon in place of wine or a cocktail. Although it is called "mineral water," this beverage is not particularly high in minerals. Dr. Walter Mertz of the Department of Agriculture says, "People may like the little bubbles dancing in their glass, but bottled water is not a bit more healthy than tap water" (91). While it is not more healthful, it is not less healthful, either. It is just a different form. And it's a good way to meet your added need for water. Different bottled waters have different flavors; some are sparkling while others are not. Many come with a flavor—lemon-lime, grapefruit, cherry, or berry—and still have zero calories.

There are a number of alternatives for those who do not drink alcoholic beverages. In addition to juice and soft drinks, many nonalcoholic beers and wines are now available. Most restaurants carry at least one choice of both nonalcoholic wine and beer. The federal government labeling standard for "nonalcoholic" is less than 0.5 percent alcohol by volume; the labeling standard for "no alcohol" is less than 0.05 percent alcohol by volume (chocolate, orange juice, and sauerkraut fall between these two percentages) (119).

You may be familiar with the Bloody Mary cocktail, spiced tomato juice mixed with vodka; a better choice during pregnancy would be the no-alcohol Virgin Mary. Or try the Mother Mary, a perfect drink for the mother-to-be: eight ounces of cold, refreshing tap or mineral water on the rocks.

WHAT WILL YOU HAVE TO DRINK?

BEVERAGE	AMOUNT	CALORIES	NUTRIENTS	COMMENT
Tap water	8 oz.	0	May have fluoride	Free and available to all
Club soda	8 oz.	0	May have sodium	Mother Nature, with added bubbles
Tomato juice, canned	8 oz.	51	Sodium, vitamin A, vitamin C, B vitamins, iron	Aids absorption of iron and other nutrients
Coffee (no cream or sugar)	6 oz.	4	Small amounts of potassium, magnesium	Contains caffeine (See page 200)
Tea	6 oz.	2	Small amounts of potassium, magnesium	Contains stimulants; may impair nutrient absorption (See page 203)
Milk, skim 1% fat 2% fat whole	8 oz.	86 102 121 157	Protein, calcium, phosphorus, riboflavin, vitamin A, vitamin D, other vitamins and minerals	A prime source of baby-building calcium; a problem only to those who are lactose-intolerant; a very protective food during pregnancy and lactation

BEVERAGE	AMOUNT	CALORIES	NUTRIENTS	COMMENT
Wine	$3\frac{1}{2}$ oz.	70–90	Traces of some minerals	Potential dangers from alcohol
Wine coolers	12 oz.	215	Traces of some minerals	Potential dangers from alcohol
Nonalcoholic wine	7 oz.	54	Traces of some minerals	Although not tested specifically for safety during pregnancy, there is no reason to believe that it is not safe
Beer	12 oz.	136–155	Carbohydrate, traces of B vitamins	Potential dangers from alcohol
Light beer	12 oz.	100–115	Carbohydrate, traces of B vitamins	Potential dangers from alcohol
Nonalcoholic beer	12 oz.	72	Traces of some minerals	Although not tested specifically for safety during pregnancy, there is no reason to believe that it is not safe

BEVERAGE	AMOUNT	CALORIES	NUTRIENTS	COMMENT
Spirits (gin, whiskey, vodka, rum, scotch, etc.)	$1\frac{1}{2}$ oz. (jigger)	120	None	Potential danger from alcohol; warning to pregnant women on labels

Multicategory Foods

A number of popular foods do not appear on the lists because they include items from more than one group. Pizza, for instance, can be evaluated in terms of its ingredients and the groups they best fit into:

Crust—bread, 1 serving per slice
Cheese—milk and dairy, 1 serving per slice
Tomato sauce—vegetable, $\frac{1}{2}$ serving per slice
Sausage—protein, $\frac{1}{2}$ serving per slice

Soups can contribute vegetables, protein foods, and dairy items. A raw spinach salad may have spinach (green leafy vegetable), mushrooms (other vegetables), tomatoes (vitamins A and C rich), hard-cooked egg (protein), and salad dressing (fats and oils).

If cooking for one or two seems a chore or if you are in a hurry, many frozen dinners are available that contain portions of foods from several Best Choice lists. Keep them on hand in your freezer. If you work outside the home and have access to a microwave oven, bring along a frozen meal for an easy and healthful lunch.

With a bit of practice, you will find you can place your food choices into the appropriate categories. Precision is not important; these lists are just a way to help you get an overall idea of the way your diet balances out. *If you are regularly neglecting a whole group of foods, chances are you are missing out on some important nutrients.*

The All-You-Can-Eat Pregnancy Myth

When you first heard that you were going to need more calories during pregnancy, didn't you think, "Oh good! Now I can eat as much as I want"? The bubble bursts, however, when you find that added calories are needed primarily to ensure adequate intake of essential nutrients, and thus must be chosen with care.

If you eat only the suggested number of servings of foods from the Best Choices food lists, you will get all the recommended nutrients, except calories. Then you can eat anything you wish, from any list, to make up the remaining calories. But the chances are by the time you increase your milk consumption and add the extra vegetable or two that is recommended during pregnancy, you will also have eaten adequate calories. Unless you're not gaining adequate weight, eating all you want remains a myth.

SURPRISE SUPERSTARS

Everyone knows that milk and orange juice are nutritious, but there are many other foods whose healthful attributes aren't widely recognized. During this time of nutritional consciousness-raising, discover these power-packed food values.

Liver

✳ Liver is the worst kept nutritional secret and the topic of endless jokes. Stop laughing and take another look, because liver is an unusually good source of almost every important nutrient. When you look through the nutrient charts you will see that liver is an excellent source of most vitamins and minerals. Give it a try. Many restaurants have liver and onions or bacon on their menu, if you don't want to prepare it yourself. Liver pâté is an elegant as well as a nutritious appetizer. How about a chicken liver omelet or a liver sausage sandwich? We like calves' liver thinly sliced and quickly sautéed with peppers, mushrooms, and onions.

Some people question eating liver because the liver can store toxins. If this concerns you, choose calves' liver (young animals have less exposure to toxins), and don't eat liver more than once a week.

If you cannot face it "straight," have your butcher grind a quarter-pound of liver with a pound of ground beef. Cook it as you usually cook ground beef. You won't even know it's there!

Greens, Kale, Broccoli

✳ These foods join spinach as great nutritional bargains. All give more than a whole day's supply of vitamins A and C, many B vitamins, and lots of minerals for less than fifty calories per serving. Get out your favorite cookbook and find ways to prepare them!

Cantaloupe

✳ Cantaloupe is not only refreshing and delicious but also a good buy when in season. Half of a medium-size cantaloupe has potassium, enough vitamins A and C for a whole day, and only sixty calories. Fill a cantaloupe wedge with cottage cheese, tuna salad, or chicken salad for a quick and easy meal.

Hearty Soups

✳ Hearty soups are good, nutritious convenience foods. Split pea or bean soups, minestrone, and chunky-style canned or frozen soups have lots of vegetables, giving a variety of nutrients including vitamin A and some protein. They require only heating. They do contain quite a bit of salt, but that should not be a problem during pregnancy. Have soup handy for when you don't feel like cooking, and enjoy a bowl with whole-grain crackers, a wedge of cheese, and a piece of fruit. Of course, hearty homemade soups are great too if you have the time.

Beans

✳ All beans are not of equal nutrient value. Wax beans and green beans are tasty but not particularly rich in nutrients. Legumes, dried beans, and peas are the very best nutritionally. You will find split peas, lentils, kidney beans, and garbanzo beans on many of our Best Sources lists of vitamins and minerals. Dried peas and beans are also excellent sources of protein, complex carbohydrate, and fiber. Virtually everything in them is good for you, and they have no cholesterol and little fat. On top of that, they are inexpensive!

Traditional preparation of most dried peas and beans requires hours of time for soaking and cooking. However, cooking pea or bean soups in a crockpot overnight or while you are at work is easy. Many people prefer buying canned or frozen lima beans and black-eyed peas. Look for canned vegetarian refried beans, prepared without lard, for making tacos and bean dip. Put canned chili and baked beans on your pantry shelf for quick meals. Garbanzo and kidney beans are frequently found at salad bars. Use beans to top salads or add to soups.

MEALTIMES

Rule number one for planning your diet during pregnancy is to *eat at regular times.* This means eating three main meals a day and two healthful snacks, or five or six smaller meals at regular intervals.

Breaking the Fast

You may not be a breakfast eater—many people are not—but breakfast is essential during pregnancy. Energy reserves run low after a long night without food, and both you and the baby need refueling. Recent studies suggest that even relatively short fasts—from midnight to noon, for instance—can make your baby hungry even if you are not. The baby's developing brain and nervous system need carbohydrate, which is best supplied by frequent meals.

Breakfast does not need to be bacon and eggs or cereal and toast. Your body has no preconceived ideas about what is appropriate for specific meals. If you feel like it, eat a grilled cheese sandwich, cottage cheese and fruit, leftover casserole, hot soup, or some tuna salad. If making breakfast seems like a lot of time and trouble to you, take advantage of quick-to-fix foods like frozen waffles, quick breakfast drinks made with milk, or ready-to-eat muffins and nut breads.

Cereals are an excellent source of vitamins, minerals, and fiber. If you choose a cereal that is not presweetened, you can control the amount of sugar (and calories) you get. Granola-type cereals, thought by many to be very healthful, often contain large amounts of sugar and some oil, and are high in calories. A half-cup serving of one popular brand contains 260 calories; a whole cup of cornflakes has only 89 calories. Granola and granola bars are good foods and nutritious snacks, however, if you are not having a problem controlling your weight.

During pregnancy it is especially important to find the extra few minutes it takes to eat breakfast. On those days when you are running late and must dash off, make it a point to take along a piece of fruit, peanut butter and crackers, a few oatmeal cookies, or a container of fruit yogurt to eat on the way.

In many offices, schools, and factories, the midmorning break is a welcome ritual. Consider alternatives to coffee and doughnuts or sweet rolls, if that's been your habit. How about a corn or bran muffin, a bagel, a piece of fresh fruit, or a glass of milk and a slice of banana bread? The calories may be as high as you would find in a sweet roll, but these foods have a higher nutrient density and contribute more to your overall nutritional needs.

Lunch

Lunch is the meal most frequently eaten away from home. Whether you brown bag it or select meals from a cafeteria or restaurant menu, there are choices to be made. Try to evaluate your food selections; even if what you have to choose from does not represent the best of all possible foods, there are always some choices that are going to be better for you than others.

PUTTING LUNCH TO THE TEST

A SAMPLE MENU	THE NUTRITIONAL CRITIQUE
Ham sandwich on white bread with mayonnaise and mustard	The sandwich is high in protein. Use less or light mayonnaise. Add some lettuce and tomato to the sandwich and order it on whole-grain bread.
Potato chips	They won't hurt you, but they won't help you much either. High in fat, salt, and calories, they contain few nutrients. Better choices to accompany your sandwich are raw vegetables, bean salad, or cole slaw.
Brownies	If having a baby means giving up brownies, we'd have a good hedge against population growth! Consider the brownie in light of your total day's intake of fat and calories. At least the nuts have fiber. A brownie for lunch means no rich dessert for

A SAMPLE MENU	THE NUTRITIONAL CRITIQUE
	dinner. Fresh fruit, on the other hand, is always a good choice for dessert and is usually available.
Cola drink	How about having your second glass of milk at lunch, or maybe a glass of tomato juice?

Dinner

There may be times when spending an hour in the kitchen is neither practical nor desirable. There are many healthy alternatives to fast-food that you can pick up quickly at a local supermarket.

10 FAST HEALTHFUL MEALS

1. Seafood-citrus salad (salad greens and grapefruit segments from salad bar topped with 2–3 oz. cooked shrimp or crabmeat from seafood counter)
   Reduced-calorie creamy cucumber dressing
   Rice cakes or sourdough breadsticks
   Lime-flavored mineral water
2. Toasted whole-grain waffles with fresh bananas and strawberries
   Mixed fruit yogurt
   Instant cocoa
3. Rotisseried chicken
   Vinegar-style cucumber salad (from deli, well drained)

Fresh orange or tangelo quarters
Whole-wheat crackers
Hot V-8 juice

4. Lean roast beef sandwich on whole-wheat bread or roll with mustard, lettuce, and tomato
   Artichokes and sweet green and red peppers (from salad bar)
   Honeydew melon wedge
   Skim milk

5. Cantaloupe half filled with cottage cheese garnished with fresh grapes
   Bran muffin with whipped margarine
   Fresh orange juice spritzer (OJ and club soda)

6. Canned or frozen lentil soup (may be thinned with water or chicken broth)
   Hearty rye bread with whipped margarine
   Kiwi fruit or fresh plums
   Skim milk

7. Sardines or canned salmon in pita pocket with onion, tomato, and lettuce
   Potato salad
   Carrot and celery sticks
   Pineapple juice

8. Sliced turkey with vegetable crudités (3 oz. sliced turkey from deli, with broccoli flowerets, cauliflower buds, cucumbers, and tomatoes from salad bar)
   Yogurt-dill dip
   Corn muffins
   Skim milk
   Oatmeal raisin cookie

9. Toasted open-faced cheese sandwich on seven-grain bread (2 oz. light Swiss, Cheddar, or Monterey Jack cheese)
   Fresh spinach topped with marinated mushroom salad or sliced mushrooms and garbanzos from salad bar with Italian dressing
   Fresh apple or pear
   Tomato juice

10. Choice of frozen dinners: light sweet & sour chicken, chicken cacciatore with spaghetti, sirloin roast with mushroom gravy, parslied potatoes, broccoli, and carrots
    No-alcohol wine
    Fresh grapes and Jarlsberg cheese wedge

The Fast-Food Fetus

About half of every food dollar in the United States today is spent eating away from home and much of this is spent in fast-food restaurants (130). Though it might cost more than twice as much as you'd pay to prepare the same food at home, fast-food is a staple in many diets.

Fast-food menus may not offer a range of foods adequate to meet all of your needs. Without fresh fruits and vegetables, they often lack vitamins A and C and folate. Fiber is noticeably absent in highly processed foods. While some may be low in sugar, most fast-foods are high in both fat and calories. But even fast-food chains are getting the message; salad bars, potato bars, grilled chicken sandwiches, fajitas, and chili are available at various fast-food chains.

The nutritional pluses of fast-food may surprise you. Lean ground beef, chicken, fish, and pizza are good sources of protein; buns, pizza crusts, and taco shells contribute complex carbohydrate. Shakes (some are not called *milk*shakes) are made from dry milk solids, and some contain saturated coconut oil, but they do supply calcium, riboflavin, niacin, and protein. Most fast food restaurants provide nutrition information, if you ask for it.

The choices you make from the fast-food menu can tip the balance of your diet. Here are some guidelines for good choices.

- Eat your burgers without the special sauces that contribute unnecessary fats and calories; scrape some of the tartar sauce off your fish sandwich.
- Add lettuce, tomato, and cheese to your burgers.
- Drink skim or 2% milk instead of a shake, soft drink, tea, or coffee. If milk is not available, the second-best choices are shakes, fruit juice (not fruit drink), lemonade, and water.
- Eat large pieces of fried fish or chicken rather than small ones that have more batter and thus retain more fat from frying. A fried chicken breast has far less fat than chicken nuggets.
- Accompany your burger with a salad or coleslaw rather than fries. Skip the gravy on the mashed potatoes that come with a chicken dinner. If corn-on-the-cob is available, order it.
- Go with the original-style chicken; extra crispy has extra calories, fat, and salt.
- Look at the fried food you eat at a fast-food restaurant as part of the day's total intake and make adjustments at other meals. It may be the day for a grapefruit half and an English muffin with breakfast and a large salad with low-fat dressing at lunch.

- Avoid more than one fried food in the same meal—do not have both fried chicken and fried potatoes.

Snacking That's Good for You

Snacks are bad for you—right? Well, yes and no. We can't offer much of a nutritional defense for snack foods that contain little more than calories and are high in sugar, salt, and fat. But if snacks help provide the essential nutrients you need, a great deal can be said for them.

Nutritious snacks are identified earlier in this chapter, designated as Best or Other choices. They include fresh fruit and raw vegetables, banana-nut bread, sunflower seeds, dried fruit, frozen fruit bars, and fruit-flavored yogurt. Some of that milk you are supposed to drink may be enjoyed as a bedtime snack with gingersnaps or graham crackers. Popcorn sprinkled with Parmesan cheese or herbs is relatively low in calories (if you skip the butter) and a good source of fiber.

The role of snacks in your diet will depend in large part on your need for calories. Women who need extra calories because of their young age or because they were underweight before becoming pregnant may find that they can add to their intake by having several expanded snacks in addition to regular meals. A milkshake, a peanut butter and jelly sandwich with a glass of milk, or a dish of cottage cheese with fruit adds both calories and nutrients.

PREGNANCY ON A BUDGET

Eating well during pregnancy is not a luxury, but an investment in your child's future that you cannot afford to neglect.

The Montreal Diet Dispensary mothers improved the outcome of their pregnancies by the mere addition of eggs, milk, and oranges. No additional food costs need be incurred if you are willing to substitute nutritious foods for some of those that contribute little to the diet. As you become more aware of the role of eating in health, you will find you are less likely to choose foods merely because you like them, because you are in the habit of buying them, or because you see them advertised.

Consider your trips to the supermarket as a part of prenatal care: "I see my doctor once a month. I go to Lamaze classes. I go to the supermarket . . ." Select foods based on several of the following criteria.

- It's good for me and the baby.
- I like it.
- The rest of my family will eat it.
- It's a good buy this week (check the food pages in the newspaper).
- I know how to prepare the food or have a recipe I'd like to try.
- It's quick and easy.

Then plan your shopping trip, and remember:

- Eat before you shop because everything looks good when you are hungry, and you may overspend.
- Select some fresh fruits and vegetables to use right away and others that will keep until the end of the week.
- Do not buy more fresh fruits and vegetables than you can use.
- Prepare a list, but be flexible. Try not to make impulse purchases.

- Avoid buying nonnutritious foods that will serve only as temptation. If all the choices in your refrigerator are good ones, you can't go wrong.
- Purchase some raw fruits and vegetables to keep on hand for munching.
- Get some nonfat dry milk in case you run out of fresh milk.
- Take time to read labels to know what you are getting for your money.
- Switch to whole-grain crackers and breads.
- Try at least one new food from the Best Choice lists each week to have a more varied diet.

Bon appétit!

4

The Proteins, Carbohydrates, and Fats of Pregnancy

QUICK QUIZ

How much do you know about carbohydrate, protein, and fat and their relationship to pregnancy? Answer these questions and then read the chapter. Correct answers are on page 293.

TRUE OR FALSE

___ 1. Carbohydrate is more fattening than protein.

___ 2. Protein foods are the best source of energy during pregnancy.

___ 3. More than half of the calories you eat should come from carbohydrate foods.

___ 4. Honey is a good source of many nutrients.

___ 5. Pregnant women should eat a meal or snack every 3 to 4 hours during the day.

___ 6. All women need at least 500 more calories a day during pregnancy.

___ 7. Applesauce is a good source of dietary fiber.

___ 8. Butter and margarine have about the same number of calories.

___ 9. Many women in the United States do not eat enough protein when they are pregnant.

___ 10. Cholesterol in foods you eat can accumulate in fetal arteries.

Those who "speak nutrition" sometimes make it as difficult to understand as a foreign language. "Grams of protein" and "calories from carbohydrate" may sound more like Greek than food. Just as the language course you take in a classroom doesn't really "take" until you find yourself in a situation where you need it in order to be understood, nutrition becomes much more meaningful when it has direct bearing on what's happening to you. During pregnancy, every meal affects you and your baby.

What is nutrition? Simply defined, it is the process by which your body uses food. In the thousands of foods you can eat or drink, there are only fifty *nutrients,* or substances that are absolutely essential. These necessary nutrients can be categorized into six groups: proteins, carbohydrates, fats, vitamins, minerals, and water.

RDAs AND U.S.RDAs

The Food and Nutrition Board of the National Academy of Sciences/National Research Council publishes suggested amounts for essential nutrients—vitamins, minerals, proteins, carbohydrates, and fats. These guidelines, called Recommended Dietary Allowances (RDAs), set specific daily nutrient intakes, based on an estimate of what the body needs to maintain health. The level that the RDA establishes for each nutrient is actually higher than the average person needs. This is because the level is determined by estimating the range of human nutritional needs, setting the RDA from the high end of the range, and adding a bit more. The built-in extra provides a margin for healthy individuals who have higher than normal needs. Think of the RDAs not as minimums but as goals for good nutrition that reflect current scientific thinking.

The RDAs are revised about every five years to accommodate advances in nutrition knowledge. The current RDAs, the tenth revised edition, were published in 1989 and include recommended levels of protein, calories, eleven vitamins, and seven minerals for daily consumption by healthy people. There are separate allowances for pregnant and lactating women. For two other vitamins and five minerals about which less is known, the Food and Nutrition Board published "estimated safe and adequate intakes."

U.S. RDAs, the United States Recommended Dietary Allowances you see on many food labels, are different from RDAs. U.S.RDAs are figures the Food and Drug Administration established based on the 1968 RDAs. They are used on food labels by processors who choose to provide nutritional information, and they represent the high end of the RDA range. Most people do not need as much of each nutrient as is suggested in the U.S.RDAs. The agencies of the federal government which label foods, the United States Department of Agriculture, and the Food and Drug Administration are in the process of completely revising the format and type of information on food labels.

The new labels are expected to present information as percentage of daily recommended values. While the new values are based on the needs of adults (not pregnant) and children over age four, they can help you identify good sources of particular nutrients. For example, a food that contains 30 percent of the daily recommended value of a specific nutrient is a very good source, whether or not you are pregnant. If you see a food label with less than 5 percent of each nutrient, you know that the food will not contribute significantly to your diet—except, perhaps, in calories.

The following chart sets goals for nutrient intake during pregnancy and lactation. In the following chapters, we will discuss the kinds of foods you can choose to meet these needs. And when we discuss individual nutrients, we will remind you of their RDA. But remember: *Nutrition is food, not numbers. You can eat well even if you do not understand the chart!*

RECOMMENDED DIETARY ALLOWANCES FOR WOMEN

	AGE 19–24	AGE 25–50	PREGNANT	LACTATING 1ST 6 MOS.	LACTATING 2ND 6 MOS.
Protein, grams	46	50	60	65	62
Vitamin A, retinol equivalents, micrograms*	800	800	800	1300	1200
Vitamin D, micrograms	10	5	10	10	10

	AGE 19–24	AGE 25–50	PREGNANT	LACTATING 1ST 6 MOS.	LACTATING 2ND 6 MOS.
Vitamin E, alpha tocopherol equivalents, milligrams*	8	8	10	12	11
Vitamin K, micrograms	60	65	65	65	65
Vitamin C, milligrams	60	60	70	95	90
Thiamin, milligrams	1.1	1.1	1.5	1.6	1.6
Riboflavin, milligrams	1.3	1.3	1.6	1.8	1.7
Niacin, niacin equivalents, milligrams*	15	15	17	20	20
Vitamin B_6, milligrams	1.6	1.6	2.2	2.1	2.1
Folate, micrograms	180	180	400	280	260
Vitamin B_{12}, micrograms	2.0	2.0	2.2	2.6	2.6
Calcium, milligrams	1200	800	1200	1200	1200

	AGE 19–24	AGE 25–50	PREGNANT	LACTATING 1ST 6 MOS.	LACTATING 2ND 6 MOS.
Phosphorus, milligrams	1200	800	1200	1200	1200
Magnesium, milligrams	280	280	320	355	340
Iron, milligrams	15	15	30	15	15
Zinc, milligrams	12	12	15	19	16
Iodine, micrograms	150	150	175	200	200
Selenium, micrograms	55	55	65	75	75

SOURCE: (174)
* See vitamin charts in chapter 5 for explanation of equivalents.

PROTEIN: THE CELL BUILDER

Living things, large and small, are made of cells. Part of every cell is protein. Throughout life, protein rebuilds cells that are destroyed because of wear and tear, infection, or surgery. Most pregnant American women eat more protein than is recommended. But it's important to understand how protein is used by the body to ensure that it is being used for baby-building and not for energy.

Protein is made up of *amino acids,* sometimes called "the

building blocks of protein." In chapter 1, we explained how amino acids pass from the mother to the fetus. Amino acids can be put together like ingredients in a recipe to make cells for tough fibrous muscle tissue, ligaments, hair, and fingernails. Amino acids combine in different ways to form protein complexes needed for bones, brain tissue, and blood. Protein is also used in the construction of the placenta and uterus, and it is in amniotic fluid that the fetus floats in and swallows. Protein is also necessary in the mother's blood supply, which must expand to carry enough oxygen for both maternal and fetal tissues.

Protein plays a key role in regulating body processes. Body regulators include enzymes, hormones, and antibodies. *Enzymes* initiate and promote chemical reactions in the body. Digestion, for example, requires many enzymes to break down food into easily absorbed nutrients. *Hormones* accelerate or slow down body processes and are especially variable during pregnancy. It has been speculated, though not proven, that the same hormones that give some women menstrual problems also cause morning sickness. Special hormones are produced by the placenta to regulate the way nutrients are used during pregnancy. *Antibodies* are the health protectors that ward off illness. At the beginning of this book, we told you about an amazing "prenatal protein vaccination" that passes intact from mother to fetus.

Protein is needed at an increasingly greater rate as pregnancy progresses. At first, it's used to prepare the mother; then it is diverted to begin baby-building. Based on protein needs to build and maintain additional tissue, and the uncertainty of the rate at which protein is deposited in these tissues, the RDA committee recommends an increase in protein throughout pregnancy (174).

All Protein Is Not Equal

The body manufactures eleven of the twenty amino acids it needs; nine must be supplied (for both you and the baby you're carrying) from foods you eat. These nine are called the *essential amino acids.* In order for your little bundle of protein to grow (or your own body to get the protein it needs), all nine must be present—all of them and at the same time.

Animal protein foods have some of each of the nine essential amino acids. Animal sources of protein are therefore called *complete proteins.* An exception is gelatin. Though it comes from an animal source, it lacks an essential amino acid and cannot, by itself, build new cells for your fingernails or your baby's tissues.

Plant proteins contain most of the essential amino acids, but are low in or missing one or two of them. These plant sources of proteins are called low quality, or low biological value or incomplete proteins. An *incomplete protein* by itself cannot be used to build or repair tissue. But if you eat plant proteins with other foods containing the missing amino acids within the same day, your body gets all the amino acids to build proteins your body and your baby need.

If you are a vegetarian, or rely heavily on plant foods for protein, you will need to take special care during pregnancy to eat foods that provide all of the essential amino acids. Vegetarians traditionally choose foods that complement each other—in other words, choosing vegetable proteins that together provide all the essential amino acids. Examples include beans with rice, cheese with noodles, peanut butter with whole-grain bread, and sesame seeds with garbanzo beans. The simple addition of milk to cereal gives the cereal grains body-building power.

SOURCES OF PROTEIN

ANIMAL PROTEIN	PLANT PROTEIN
Dairy products (milk, cheese, yogurt)	Grains (rice, corn, wheat)
Eggs	Legumes (beans, soybeans)
Fish	Nuts and seeds
Meat	Tofu and other soy products
Poultry	Vegetables (green peas, broccoli)

If you are a committed vegetarian, you may be very knowledgeable about mixing and matching to obtain complete proteins; but if you are a casual vegetarian who doesn't eat meat or drink milk, your diet may need to be improved for pregnancy.

If you are a strict vegetarian and eat no dairy products or eggs, consult a registered dietitian or your doctor about the adequacy of your diet for pregnancy. Chances are they will have to devise a plan to ensure you get enough calories, protein, vitamins, and minerals.

How Much Protein?

The protein RDA for pregnancy is sixty grams per day. This is ten grams more than a nonpregnant woman of twenty-five to fifty needs and fourteen grams more than a woman of nineteen to twenty-four needs. Because there are several different ways to estimate nutritional requirements, and each has limitations, nutrition experts do not always agree with the RDA—or with each other. In 1990, the Subcommittee on Dietary Intake and Nutrient Supplement During Pregnancy reviewed all the data and concluded that while the RDAs are useful in evaluating the average nutrient intakes of pregnant women, recommendations must be based on an assessment of individual needs.

The average pregnant female in the United States eats from 75 to 110 grams of protein a day—well over the recommended 1989 RDAs (174). Nevertheless, eating more than the RDA levels of protein is no guarantee of meeting your protein needs. The RDAs assume that much of protein eaten is from animal sources, which are complete proteins. Since more protein is needed if all of it comes from vegetable sources, vegetarians will need somewhat more than the RDA of 60 grams.

Protein status is also influenced by calorie intake. Inadequate calorie intake can cause protein deficiency. You must get enough calories from nonprotein foods (carbohydrate and fat) or your body will use the protein you ingest for energy rather than building cells. If your body has a choice between producing energy and building cells, its first priority is energy. The most available source of energy is glucose, which enters the bloodstream when carbohydrate foods are digested and absorbed. Carbohydrate foods are able to maintain blood glucose levels for only three to four hours after they are eaten. Regular meals and snacks that include carbohydrates replenish blood glucose levels. If the level of blood glucose drops, body fat and proteins are broken down and used for energy. But fat does not break down to glucose, so the body turns to protein to use because its structure can be broken down to make glucose as an immediate energy source. *Protein can be converted to fuel for energy, but nothing can do the job of cell-building but protein.* This is why, during pregnancy, you will want to have enough calories, primarily from carbohydrates at regular intervals, to save the protein for baby-building.

Protein foods such as meat, milk, legumes, and whole grains are valuable sources of other nutrients, and are therefore good choices to meet the demands of pregnancy.

A highly controversial practice is the use of protein supplements (powders and beverages) to prevent pregnancy-induced hypertension. The effectiveness of such use has not been demonstrated (202), and it is not recommended by the Institute of Medicine Subcommittee on Dietary Intake and Nutrient Supplements During Pregnancy (172).

PROTEIN IN FOOD

RDA in pregnancy: 60 grams per day

RDA in lactation: first 6 months, 65 grams per day

	PORTION	GRAMS OF PROTEIN	CALORIES
Cottage cheese, lowfat	1 cup	30	203
Chicken, broiled, skinless, some bone	$3\frac{1}{2}$ oz.	29	173

	PORTION	GRAMS OF PROTEIN	CALORIES
Turkey, roasted breast, skinless	3 oz.	25	135
Tuna, water packed	3 oz.	25	111
Beef: lean sirloin, broiled	3 oz.	25	180
hamburger, broiled	1 med.	20	253
Fish, halibut, broiled	3 oz.	23	119
Pork chop, panfried	1 med. (4 oz.)	18	257
Chili, beef and beans	1 cup	15	235
Ravioli with meat sauce, canned	1 cup	11	284
Taco, beef	1 med.	11	187
Tofu, bean curd	½ cup	10	94
Split pea with ham soup	1 cup	10	189
Garbanzo beans, canned	1 cup	12	285
Peanuts, dry roasted	¼ cup (1½ oz.)	9	246
Peanut butter	2 tbsp.	8	186
Milk, skim, 1%, 2%, whole	1 cup	8	86–150
Oatmeal, quick cooked	⅔ cup	5	109

	PORTION	GRAMS OF PROTEIN	CALORIES
Pumpkin seeds, roasted	1 oz.	7	148
Bologna, beef	2 oz.	6	144
Egg, boiled	1 large	6	79
Almonds, roasted	1 oz.	5	167
Spaghetti, cooked, no sauce	1 cup	5	159
Peas	½ cup	4	59
Potato, baked	1 med.	5	220
Rice	1 cup	4	186
Chicken noodle soup	1 cup	3	60
Broccoli, cooked	1 cup	5	45
Tomato soup	1 cup	2	106
Ice cream, regular vanilla	½ cup	2	134
Cornflakes	1 cup	2	110
Bread, white	1 slice	2	64
Carrots, raw	1 med.	1	31

CALORIES AND THE ENERGY BALANCE

If we say "calories," do you think "weight"? When we say "calories," we want you to think "needs"—how many calories do you need for both you and your baby to thrive? And what kind of calories do you need to provide for both energy and growth?

Your calorie needs for energy are based on three things: *basal metabolism, thermic response,* and *physical activity.*

Your caloric need for basal metabolism is the amount of energy you need to support basic body functions, like breathing and circulation. (Basal calories do not include calories used to digest food or provide energy for activities.) The more you weigh, the greater your basal metabolic rate. As you gain weight during pregnancy, you need more calories. Larger pregnant women need proportionately more calories than do smaller pregnant women. You also need calories to support the additional demands of pregnancy, such as pumping a greatly expanded blood volume.

Pregnant women who engage in weight-bearing exercise like walking or jogging should increase calories in proportion to time spent in these activities (172). Regardless of activity or age, extra energy is required for growth and maintenance of the fetus, placenta, and maternal tissues. Teenaged women need extra calories for their own growth. Fetal energy demands are greatest between the tenth and thirtieth weeks, when maternal fat is being stored (172). In the third trimester, calories are shifted to meet the rapid growth demands of the baby. Inadequate calorie intake, especially during this third trimester, may reduce the baby's birth weight (172).

Most pregnant women need about twenty-five hundred calories a day. Experts estimate that the total additional energy cost of pregnancy is fifty-five thousand to eighty-five thousand calories, (172; 174; 197) an average of three hundred calories a day above a nonpregnant woman's needs. Unless a woman begins pregnancy underweight, the National Research Council Committee notes, the additional calories are probably not necessary during the first trimester (174).

This is good because many women are not particularly hungry, and frequently suffer from morning sickness in the first trimester. The Institute of Medicine's Subcommittee on Maternal Nutrition and Weight Gain During Pregnancy notes that while the twenty-five-hundred-calorie-per-day suggestion is consistent with the higher total weight gain now being encouraged, recommendations should be based on individual assessment.

Energy needs differ from one woman to another (202). Whether or not you're pregnant, you'll put on excess weight if you consume more calories than you need. If your rate of weight gain is appropriate to your stage of pregnancy, you can assume your energy supply is adequate.

CARBOHYDRATES: THE PRIMARY SOURCE OF CALORIES

Health-conscious eaters know that carbohydrates—fruits, vegetables, and whole grains—are the staff of life. The American Dietetic Association recommends two to four servings of fruits, three to five servings of vegetables, and six or more servings of bread or grain products a day for adults (1).

Restricting carbohydrates can be very dangerous, especially during pregnancy. Fortunately, low-carbohydrate diets (such as the Atkins, Stillman, and Scarsdale diets) have gone out of fashion. But just in case you're considering limiting breads, potatoes, starches, and cereals as a way of restricting weight gain when you are pregnant, we offer the following warning: A low-carbohydrate diet can be a serious threat to an unborn child. Only glucose, the energy source from carbohydrate, can be used for development of the baby's nervous system. A limited amount of glucose can be converted from the breakdown of protein, but this isn't enough for optimal growth. When protein is used for energy, it cannot do its job of tissue building. If fat reserves are broken down for energy because you aren't eating enough carbohydrates, acids form that can be harmful to the fetus.

Your body runs twenty-four hours a day and needs a continuous supply of fuel to keep it going (the basal metabolic rate we mentioned earlier). Even when you're sleeping, your heart continues to beat and you continue to breathe. In addition, during pregnancy, your baby is on a round-the-clock growing program that burns up energy at about twice the rate of your own body.

Where does the extra energy come from? There are four potential sources: fat, protein, carbohydrate, and alcohol. Vitamins and minerals have no calories. At nine calories a gram, fat is the most concentrated source of energy. And, while there are no studies to suggest that pregnant women should reduce fat intake, we do not suggest that you eat *more* fat. Most women in the United States get more than enough protein, which has four calories per gram, and only a modest increase in protein is necessary during pregnancy. Certainly alcohol, which is correlated with birth defects, is not a recommended source of calories, especially during pregnancy. The only remaining source of calories is carbohydrate. Carbohydrate provides four calories a gram. Many carbohydrate foods are packed with vitamins, minerals, and fiber and are low in fat. Usually abundant and relatively inexpensive, carbohydrate-rich foods are the fuel of human life.

Carbohydrate in food is converted by digestion into glucose, which is easily absorbed into the bloodstream and soon on the way to performing its many tasks. Fortunately, we don't have to eat constantly to provide the steady flow of energy. Simple-sugar carbohydrates (fruits and sweets) are converted to glucose very rapidly and can be used to meet immediate energy needs. The more complex starches (grains, potatoes, corn) take longer to be broken down and therefore provide glucose over an extended period of time.

Some glucose can be stored in the liver and muscles, but it must be converted to glycogen, the body's form of starch. Glycogen breaks down to release sugar needed to maintain blood sugar levels when you have not eaten in a few hours. But just so much glycogen can be stored—usually enough to get you through the night. In the morning, it's time to eat and restore the body's carbohydrate level. Throughout the day, you need to eat regular meals and snacks.

Three Types of Carbohydrate: Sugar, Starch, and Fiber

This section is going to get technical, but if you can follow along, it will not only help you understand *why* you should eat carbs but prepare you for the inevitable day when your child wants you to help with a homework assignment about photosynthesis.

In contrast to plants, humans cannot synthesize nutrients (except vitamin D) from sunlight; we need to use plants as intermediaries. Here is how this happens:

Some of the energy the sun gives to plants is trapped within the plant and stored as glucose (like solar-heated water stored in tanks). When the plant is eaten, enzymes dissolve the bonds holding the glucose molecules together and the plant's energy enters cells to be released to provide human energy (as the hot water is dispersed to heat your home).

Because of its chemical structure, glucose is classified as a simple carbohydrate, or simple sugar. Sometimes the atoms of glucose are rearranged to become other forms of simple sugars such as fructose in front and galactose in milk. Simple sugars are found in fruits such as bananas, cherries, and berries, and in honey. The scientific word for sugar is *saccharide.* Single sugar units are called *monosaccharides.* Two simple sugars can be joined together to form double sugars. Double sugars are called *disaccharides:* Maltose is a combination of two glucose units; lactose, found in milk, is a combination of the simple sugars galactose and glucose. If fructose and glucose are bonded together, they form *sucrose.* Sucrose on your breakfast table is known as sugar. It is derived primarily from sugarcane or sugar beets.

As plants mature, they build up stores of excess energy in seeds, plant stems, leaves, bark, and roots. Since glucose is not stable enough to endure this storage process, it is transformed into a more durable form. The stored glucose is called *starch.* Going back to our home-heating analogy, starch would be a solar-energy battery. Whereas sugars are simple carbohydrates, starch is classified as a complex carbohydrate, chemically a *polysaccharide.* Polysaccharides are many sugar units linked together to form larger molecules.

Plant starch is a major source of carbohydrate in our diets. It is available in plants such as potatoes, wheat, corn, and rice. Because starch molecules are encased in a tough skin, we usually cook starch-containing foods before we eat them to soften the cell walls. Our bodies cannot absorb starch because it is a large molecule. So the process of digestion breaks down the starch into basic glucose units which are absorbed and broken down in the cells of the body to meet our energy needs.

Some of the glucose units in plants are linked together in such a way that they cannot be broken down by human enzymes. These glucose chains are called *cellulose.* Cellulose, because it is not digested and absorbed, provides no calories, but it is a source of *fiber,* or *roughage,* in our diets. Fiber passes through the digestive tract with relatively little breakdown. Along the way, fiber absorbs water and swells to give a sensation of fullness. If you have an insatiable appetite (a common symptom of pregnancy), you may find some satisfaction from eating low-calorie fiber-rich foods like raw vegetables and fresh fruit. Dried fruits, nuts, and seeds have more calories along with their fiber, but also provide extra vitamins and minerals.

Fiber is especially important during pregnancy because it helps prevent constipation and hemorrhoids. Fruits, vegetables, and grains contain different forms of fiber, each of which can be useful in keeping your body running smoothly. *Pectins* and *gums* are soft, sticky forms of fiber that are partially digestible and have unique health benefits. They are called soluble fibers. Barley, kidney beans, and apples are examples of foods containing soluble fiber. This type of fiber helps control blood-sugar levels and reduce cholesterol levels in the bloodstream. (Cholesterol isn't a major concern during pregnancy, however. See page 115.)

Foods containing bran, including bran cereals, are excellent sources of fiber and useful in digestion and elimination processes. But too much bran or other fiber can limit absorption of some vitamins and minerals. The RDA subcommittee recommends plenty of fruits, vegetables, legumes, and whole-grain cereals rather than fiber supplements (174).

There's no specific recommendation for fiber during pregnancy, but you can use the "floating feces" guide. If you're consuming enough fiber, you'll produce "floaters" that contain water and humuslike material; if your diet is fiber-poor, the process of elimination will yield "sinkers." If your diet contains few fiber-rich foods, we suggest you increase them moderately at first, and let your system adjust gradually to the change. Drink plenty of liquids along with the fiber.

Good Sources of Dietary Fiber

BREAD

Bran muffins
Cornbread
Cracked-wheat bread
Crackers with seeds
Dark whole-grain and seeded bread
Rye crackers
Whole-grain crackers
Whole-wheat bread

GRAINS

Barley
Brown rice
Buckwheat groats
Bulgur
Popcorn
Wheat germ

VEGETABLES

All raw vegetables
Brussels sprouts
Cabbage
Corn
Greens, cooked
Parsnips
Peas

FRUITS

Apples with skin
Avocado
Berries, all types
Dried apricots
Figs
Grapes
Guavas

VEGETABLES

Potato, baked
Spinach
Squash, winter

FRUITS

Nectarines
Papayas
Pears with skin
Prunes
Pumpkins
Raisins

CEREALS

Bran (all types)
Cornmeal, corn bran
Grape-Nuts
Oatmeal, oat cereals
Rice bran
Shredded wheat

NUTS & SEEDS

All

LEGUMES

Baked beans
Black-eyed peas
Garbanzos
Kidney beans
Lentils
Lima beans
Navy beans
Refried beans
Split peas

BAKED GOODS

Fig bars
Oatmeal raisin cookies
Pumpkin pie

Natural Versus Refined Carbohydrates

We have identified three types of carbohydrate: sugar, starch, and fiber. But there is another distinction to be made—between naturally available and refined, or processed, carbohydrate. *Natural carbohydrates* are found in foods as they grow. Not only are they a source of energy, but they are generally accompanied by vitamins and minerals. Fruits, vegetables, and grains contain natural carbohydrates.

Refined, or processed, carbohydrates are extracted from natural sources such as sugarcane or sugar beets. These sweet-tasting substances increase palatability, make foods brown evenly during baking, and contribute to texture. On the other hand, most highly sweetened processed foods contribute little more than calories to your diet. A startling 11 percent of total energy intake in this country is estimated to be added sweeteners, mostly sucrose and high-fructose corn syrup (174) in foods like soft drinks, candy, and Jell-O.

If you frequently eat foods with added sugar, your other food choices will have to be especially wise to provide all of the vitamins, minerals, and protein you now need.

When you read a food label, look at the ingredient list to find out if sweeteners have been added. Since ingredients are listed by weight, you can generally tell if there is a lot or only a little added sweetener. Look to see if the sweetener is listed low on the ingredient list. If a sweetener is listed first on the ingredient list, you know there is more sweetener than anything else in the food!

Sweeteners

Acesulfame K* (Sunette®)	Dextrin
Aspartame* (NutraSweet®)	Dextrose
	Fructose
Brown sugar	Glucose
Confectioners' sugar	High-fructose corn syrup
Corn syrup	Honey
Corn syrup solids	Invert sugar
Cyclamates*	Maltose

Sweeteners

Mannitol
Mannose
Maple sugar
Maple syrup
Powdered sugar
Saccharin*
Sorbitol
Sorghum
Sucrose
Table sugar
Turbinado sugar
Xylitol

* Sugar substitutes.

Sugar Versus Honey

Some people believe that white sugar is bad for you and that honey and raw sugar are healthier. Neither is true. The basic difference between white sugar, raw sugar, and honey is flavor, not nutritional value. None offers much of anything except calories. What is called "raw sugar" is, in fact, turbinado sugar. Turbinado sugar is purified like refined white sugar, but not all of the molasses has been removed. The molasses contains small amounts of iron and B vitamins. Honey, a combination of glucose and fructose, has traces of a few vitamins and minerals. Given the small amount of turbinado sugar or honey we eat, little can be said for either as a source of nutrients. Honey is an expensive source of calories. If you like the taste, enjoy it, but don't believe that it has health benefits. In fact, honey can carry spores of bacteria that cause botulism and should not be given to babies. Nonnutritive sweeteners such as aspartame and saccharin are discussed in chapter 7.

NUTRIENTS IN SUGAR AND HONEY

	SUGAR (1 TBSP.)	HONEY (1 TBSP.)
Calories	46	64
Carbohydrate (gm)	11.9	17.3
Protein (gm)	0	0.1
Calcium (mg)	0	1
Iron (mg)	0	0.1
Vitamin C (mg)	0	0

How Much Carbohydrate?

There is no specific number of grams of carbohydrate recommended as an RDA because the amount of carbohydrate depends on caloric needs which are highly variable. But the RDA subcommittee does recommend that more than half of the energy needed by everyone beyond infancy come from carbohydrates (174). Other sources specify carbohydrates from starches and other naturally occurring sugars (like milk and fruit), and little from refined sugars.

Chapter 3 presents a balanced plan that will guide you in selecting the best carbohydrate sources. Carbohydrate is nature's bargain nutrient. In order to get your money's worth, choose carbs that give you the extras along with the calories.

FAT: THE GREAT PROTECTOR

When you're pregnant, your body converts fat to help meet its nonstop needs for energy and to build up reserves for emergencies and for the increasing demands for energy that lie ahead. At nine calories per gram, fat is the most concentrated source of calories. Women who are underweight may be advised to eat more fat-containing foods—the risks of inadequate weight gain outweigh the risks of heart disease or other potential problems associated with fat. Blood tests show higher levels of all types of fat and cholesterol during pregnancy, but this is considered normal (197).

The added weight and bulk created by extra body fat may be difficult for you to accept. But it is nature's way of protecting your baby in the critical period before birth, during labor and delivery, and during breast-feeding. Fat in your breasts protects the mammary glands; a pad of fat under kidneys cushions them when you walk and protects them if you fall; a layer of insulating fat under your skin keeps you and your baby warm in cold weather and protects both of you from injuries.

In the absence of enough calories, particularly from carbohydrates, the body has to use dietary or stored fat for energy. But the type of energy from fat cannot be used by the brain or nerves. When excess fat is burned for energy, a fat by-product called ketones is produced. Ketones are potentially toxic because they increase the concentration of acid in the blood. We don't really know what this may do during normal pregnancy, but we do know that severe cases of ketosis in pregnant women with diabetes can be harmful to fetal development (33). Limiting calories from carbohydrates by dieting or skipping meals, especially during the last trimester, can harm the baby.

The fetus demands small amounts of *linoleic acid,* a component of fat, for development of brain cells and the central nervous system. Linoleic acid cannot be produced by the body. The need for dietary linoleic acid was discovered when premature babies fed nonfat formulas developed severe skin problems (85). Most adult women who eat as little as two tablespoons of oil or fat in a day get enough linoleic acid to meet their own needs and those imposed by pregnancy.

Most women do not have to be concerned about cholesterol during pregnancy. Cholesterol is necessary for the production of placental hormones and your baby's brain tissues. Unless your doctor specifically wants you to limit cholesterol, you need not be overly cautious about it during pregnancy. Nor do you have to seek out foods containing cholesterol; your body can manufacture all the cholesterol you'll need before, during, and after pregnancy.

Several high-cholesterol foods are recommended during pregnancy because they provide important nutrients. Liver is a nutritional bonanza. Eggs are an easy-to-prepare and economical source of high-quality protein, many vitamins, and minerals. Don't limit these foods during pregnancy unless you have a medical reason to do so.

Fat Rations

Various health organizations, including the American Dietetic Association, National Cancer Institute, and the American Heart Association, have recommended a diet that provides no more than 30 percent of calories from fat for adults. There are no studies that indicate whether this standard should be applied during pregnancy. Though we recognize the value of fat in the diet of pregnant women, we do not advocate unlimited fat. A high-fat diet may further elevate your blood cholesterol and fats that are already at elevated levels during pregnancy. A very low-fat diet, on the other hand, may accelerate the breakdown of fat deposits and increase the production of fat by your liver to meet the physiological needs of pregnancy. Neither is desirable (197). We advocate nutrient-rich foods with moderate amounts of fat. Generally, a pregnant woman eating 2200 calories a day should try not to exceed a total of 73 grams of fat per day; if 2500 calories are eaten, a maximum of 83 grams of fat may be eaten. This is equivalent to 30 percent of calories from fat, the general recommendation for moderate intake.

Here are some ways to reduce the fat in your diet.

Choose low-fat foods
Eat smaller portions of high-fat foods
Have high-fat foods less frequently
Balance what you eat during the day: If you want to splurge at dinner, have a cottage cheese and fruit plate at lunch
Cut back on fried foods
Substitute fat-reduced foods (margarine, salad dressing, cheese)
Eat more carbohydrates
Use fewer sauces and gravies
Be aware of not just how much but what kind of fat you eat
Read labels and choose lower-fat foods.

Types of Fat

Fat is classified as *saturated* and *unsaturated* (*monounsaturated* and *polyunsaturated*). Usually, animal fats (butter, lard, beef) are more saturated than vegetable fats (corn, nuts). And generally, the more solid a fat is, the more saturated it is. Solid vegetable margarine, for instance, is more saturated than liquid vegetable oil. Ironically, the most saturated fats are found in coconut, palm, and palm kernel oil, which are sometimes used in commercial baked products. The new format for nutrition labeling will tell you the total amount of fat and the grams of saturated fat in each food you buy. Look for ones with less total fat, and fewer grams of saturated fat.

FATS IN FOOD

FOOD	PORTION	GRAMS FAT	CALORIES
Fast-food fish sandwich w/bun and sauce	1	23	431
Beef, hamburger	3.5 oz.	19	275
Ice cream, rich (16% fat)	6 oz.	18	262
Peanut butter	2 tbsp.	16	190
Fast-food hamburger w/bun, $\frac{1}{4}$ lb. meat	1	15	396
Nuts, mixed	1 oz.	15	169
Avocado	$\frac{1}{2}$ med.	15	153

FOOD	PORTION	GRAMS FAT	CALORIES
Chocolate bar (Hershey's)	1.6 oz.	15	254
Oils: corn, safflower, peanut	1 tbsp.	14	120
French fries, fast-food	3 oz.	13	227
Frankfurter (no bun)	1 med.	13	142
Bologna	2 oz.	13	174
French dressing	2 tbsp.	13	134
Danish pastry	$2\frac{1}{2}$ oz.	12	249
Butter	1 tbsp.	12	108
Margarine	1 tbsp.	11	102
Mayonnaise	1 tbsp.	11	100
Ice cream, regular (10% fat)	6 oz.	11	200
Cream cheese	1 oz./2 tbsp.	10	99
Bacon, crisp	3 strips	9	109
Milk, whole	1 cup	9	157
Corn chips	1 oz.	9	153
Cream of mushroom soup	1 cup	9	129
Ham	3 oz.	9	155
Cheese: American, Swiss, Muenster, Gouda	1 oz.	8	105
Tuna, oil packed	3 oz.	7	169
Beef, lean sirloin	3 oz.	7	178
Egg, boiled	1 lg	6	79
Milk, 2%	1 cup	5	120
Sour cream	2 tbsp.	5	52

FOOD	PORTION	GRAMS FAT	CALORIES
Creamed cottage cheese	4 oz.	5	117
Chicken, light meat, broiled, w/o skin	3 oz.	4	148
Frozen yogurt (regular)	6 oz.	4	157
Milk, 1%	1 cup	3	104
Chicken noodle soup	1 cup	2	58
Tuna, water packed	3 oz.	1	111
Fish, broiled	3 oz.	1	109
Milk, skim	1 cup	0–1	86
Most fresh fruits and vegetables	1 serving	0	variable

Saturated fat in foods, even more than cholesterol in foods, raises blood cholesterol levels. Most Americans eat too much saturated fat. Health organizations say eating equal amounts of each of the three types of fat is the best approach. This is hard to track on a day-to-day basis, but if you eat less total fat while concentrating on reducing saturated fat, you're likely to come out about right. Labels will tell you amounts and often types of fat in specific foods. If you follow the advice in chapter 3 and emphasize the Best Choice foods in meal planning, you will eat a reasonable amount and variety of fat. The most important consideration during pregnancy is *calories,* but ideally, these calories should be supplied from a diet that provides lots of carbohydrate, enough protein, and some fat.

5
Mighty Vitamins

QUICK QUIZ

How much do you know about vitamins? Choose the one correct response. Answers are on page 293.

1. The best source of vitamin C is

   a. Slice of bread
   b. Glass of milk
   c. Hamburger patty
   d. Green pepper

2. The vitamin formed by sunlight on skin is

   a. Vitamin A
   b. Vitamin C
   c. Vitamin D
   d. Niacin

3. Treating skin problems with which vitamin-based medication is dangerous during pregnancy?

   a. Vitamin C
   b. Vitamin A
   c. Vitamin E
   d. Vitamin K

4. Milk is an important source of

   a. Vitamin D
   b. Folate
   c. Vitamin C
   d. Vitamin E

5. A deficiency of which vitamin can cause a type of anemia?

   a. Vitamin A
   b. Riboflavin
   c. Thiamin
   d. Folate

TRUE OR FALSE

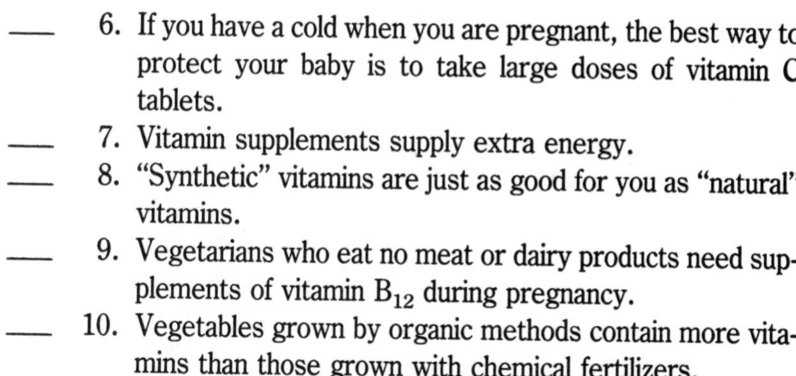

___ 6. If you have a cold when you are pregnant, the best way to protect your baby is to take large doses of vitamin C tablets.

___ 7. Vitamin supplements supply extra energy.

___ 8. "Synthetic" vitamins are just as good for you as "natural" vitamins.

___ 9. Vegetarians who eat no meat or dairy products need supplements of vitamin B_{12} during pregnancy.

___ 10. Vegetables grown by organic methods contain more vitamins than those grown with chemical fertilizers.

Remember the old word-association game, where I say a word and you respond immediately with whatever comes to mind? If I say "nutrition," there's a good chance your response would be "vitamins."

It's no wonder! Many of us grew up hearing that vitamins would make us strong and healthy. Now, posters in supermarkets and print and television ads extol the wonders of vitamins. In addition to fruits and vegetables and other vitamin-rich foods, we're offered vitamin-enriched cereal, bread, juice, pasta—even soft drinks. And just to make sure we get enough, there are a multitude of multivitamins from which to choose in supermarkets, drugstores, and health food stores as well as through direct mail and magazine advertising. Even cosmetic stores and department stores sell vitamins.

THE SPECIAL ROLE OF VITAMINS IN PREGNANCY

Will Vitamins Give Me Energy When I Feel Tired?

Vitamins are nutrients essential for life and growth—but they have no calories and thus do not supply energy to the body. They function more like a spark plug—without them, nothing works. Vitamin pills cannot replace food. Just as a car cannot run on spark-plug power alone, you cannot function on vitamins alone. To run a body, you need fuel and raw materials from the carbohydrate, protein, and fat in foods you eat.

If you are one of the very few individuals who happen to be deficient in one of the vitamins necessary to *release* energy from glucose (thiamin, for example), you may be tired; replacement of the missing nutrient may alleviate the fatigue.

Does Every Woman Need Vitamin Supplements During Pregnancy?

The Subcommittee on Dietary Intake and Nutrient Supplement During Pregnancy maintains that healthy American women should be encouraged to get the vitamins they need from foods rather than supplements. The subcommittee points out that there is a much greater risk of adverse interaction between nutrients or potential overdoses from supplements than from foods. Except for the mineral iron (discussed in chapter 6), the subcommittee recommends routine supplements only if intake is likely to be low enough to interfere with either the mother's or baby's well-being (172). The report of the RDA subcommittee concurs with this recommendation.

Other professional groups, such as the American Dietetic Association (ADA), stress that individual recommendations regarding supplements and diet should come from a physician or registered dietitian and should be based on an evaluation of dietary intake. ADA points out that women who are pregnant or breast-feeding need more of certain nutrients, particularly iron, folic acid, and calcium (1). Women who are carrying more than one baby, pregnant adolescents, substance abusers, and vegetarians are very likely to benefit from supplements (172).

We think pregnant women are well-advised to take a balanced prenatal supplement in the prescribed amount because there is little if any risk, and some potential benefit.

Recent surveys show that about 90 percent of pregnant women take vitamin or mineral supplements (172). Most physicians routinely prescribe a prenatal supplement that includes the vitamin folate (also called folic acid and folacin) because surveys have shown that many women in the U.S. have low levels of folate (196). In addition, there is evidence that oral contraceptives interfere with folate absorption (163). Some evidence suggests that use of folate supplements before conception and during early pregnancy may provide some protection against neural tube defects such as spina bifida (123). Although data are not conclusive on this issue, some experts maintain that routine supplementation of folate may be wise and without risk—before and during pregnancy (197).

The subcommittee, however, questions whether fetal needs for folate are as great as previously believed (172). They contend that healthy women who eat fruits, vegetables, and whole-grain breads and cereals can, in fact, get adequate folate (172).

A generic form of vitamin-mineral capsule with no more than 100 percent of RDA is an economical substitute. So is a fortified cereal—some contain the equivalent of a vitamin pill wrapped around flakes. Remember, though, that most capsules don't provide all of the vitamins and minerals you need, particularly calcium, so diet remains important.

The bottom line is that you should make every effort to get adequate vitamins during pregnancy by eating a variety of nutrient-rich foods. A physician or registered dietitian can evaluate your diet and discuss special problems or conditions that might affect your nutritional status. If your physician prescribes a prenatal vitamin-mineral supplement, make sure that it does not exceed the RDAs for pregnancy. Prenatal supplements are formulated to be safe for pregnancy when taken in the prescribed dosage. Single nutrients, especially vitamins in high doses, may have negative effects. These are mentioned on the charts later in this chapter in the column Dangers of Too Much. Do not take any other vitamin-mineral supplements without your doctor's advice.

Do Women Who Were on the Pill Need Special Supplements?

Whether or not women who have been taking birth-control pills need supplements depends on what type of contraceptives they used and how long they used them. If you used oral contraceptives containing high levels of estrogen (e.g., one hundred grams of mestranol or ethinyl estradiol) for more than thirty months, you may have decreased your vitamin B_6 levels and require supplementation (172). Using this type of oral contraceptive for a short period of time, however, does not suggest a need for supplementation (172).

No data are available on how low-dose estrogen (twenty to thirty-five milligrams per day) oral contraceptives affect vitamin B_6 reserves (172).

Can Vitamins Be Dangerous?

The answer quite simply is *yes!*

Excessive amounts (megadoses) of vitamins can be very dangerous to both you and your baby during pregnancy. Your baby can "overdose" if large amounts of some vitamins become concentrated in the fetal bloodstream. The baby can build up a vitamin tolerance and then suffer withdrawal symptoms when levels are reduced after birth. If you routinely take large amounts of vitamin supplements, use vitamin C when you have a cold, or use vitamin A medications for acne, read the Dangers of Too Much section of the charts at the end of this chapter. Do not risk exposing your baby to vitamin therapies that are potentially harmful.

Large doses of vitamins may be indicated for treatment of specific disease conditions, but they should be taken only under medical supervision. Vitamins prescribed for therapeutic reasons should be considered drugs, not nutrients.

In his undergraduate years, Mary's brother Fred was "into" fruits, vegetables, and nuts. During one period freshly squeezed carrot juice formed a major part of his diet. Carrot juice is an excellent source of carotene, a form of vitamin A and also an orange pigment.

One evening Fred appeared at Mary's door after driving cross-country. He was a nice shade of *peach!* At first Mary thought he had jaundice, until she looked more carefully. He had a curious problem called *xanthosis cutis,* which occurs when fat-containing cells pick up carotene pigment. He had not even noticed it because he had "oranged" gradually. Mary evaluated his diet, and he gave up his juices and returned to a more normal and varied eating pattern. It took about a month for Fred to fade.

This condition can also afflict infants who are given frequent feedings of carrots, squash, and sweet potato. Unlike a massive dose of supplementary vitamin A, the carotene in food does no permanent damage. *Toxicity is unlikely if you get your vitamins from food,* even if you eat large amounts of one food.

Are "Natural" Vitamin Supplements Better than "Synthetic" Vitamin Supplements?

Health-conscious Americans tend to rank vitamins right up there with the flag and apple pie. It comes as a shock to find that *all vitamins are chemicals.*

Each vitamin has a specific chemical structure, and these chemical configurations can be duplicated in laboratories. In order to be vitamin C, a substance must contain molecules arranged in a specific pattern; otherwise, it is not vitamin C. Thus, vitamin C is vitamin C, whether it is found in an orange or in a capsule. The advantage of the food form is that the orange has fiber, carbohydrate, fluid, other vitamins, and minerals.

Claims have been made that natural vitamin supplements are less likely to cause allergic reactions than synthetic ones, but there are no clinical data to support this. Your body cannot tell (but your wallet can) whether a supplement you consume comes from a natural source or a laboratory. The term *natural* on a vitamin label conveys no real advantages.

Do Organically Grown Foods Contain More Vitamins than Foods Grown Commercially?

There are some who believe that organically grown food is more nutritious than other food because modern farming techniques have depleted the soil and reduced the nutrient content of fruits and vegetables grown there. Studies show that the nutrient content of food is the same, whether it is grown in rich or poor soil. A carrot may be smaller if grown in poor soil, or the crop may be meager, but by weight, it still has the same nutrients. When carrots from various sources are laboratory tested using the latest technology, it cannot be determined which carrots were grown by commercial or organic/natural methods. Many studies show that nutrient values and amounts of chemical residues are comparable (40).

Government agencies control the cleanliness and safety of packaged food products, and of fresh meat, fish, poultry, eggs, and dairy products. The use of chemical pesticides on fruits and vegetables is also monitored. But there are no legal definitions of the terms *natural* and *organic* at this time, and no widespread inspection system exists to attest to the validity of claims. Food-labeling changes planned for implementation over the next few years are likely to create legal criteria that foods must meet to be labeled organic or natural. Currently, any producer can make these claims.

Consumers concerned about the nutritional value and safety of our food supply put pressure on producers to provide healthful products. It can take months for an industry to recover from unfavorable publicity. We'll talk more about food additives and food safety in chapter 7.

VITAMIN ESSENTIALS

The charts that follow highlight points that are especially important for you during your pregnancy. Use the charts as a reference when you have questions about vitamins.

We've included the following information in the charts.

- *Other names:* By becoming familiar with the varied terminology used to identify vitamins, you can begin to sort fact from fiction. For instance, if you read about the wonders of pyridoxine, you will find that pyridoxine is another name for vitamin B_6. You'll also be more nutrition literate about what's on labels: ascorbic acid is vitamin C; riboflavin is a B vitamin.

Originally, all the B vitamins were thought to be one vitamin, but as more was learned, individual types were differentiated—thus, B_1 (thiamin), B_2 (niacin), B_3 (riboflavin), B_6 (pyridoxine), and B_{12}. Some substances once thought to be vitamins were later found not to be and were deleted from the list; thus, there is no B_9 or B_{11}.

- *Physical characteristics:* Vitamins are often known by the way they are absorbed and stored. Vitamins are classified as *fat-soluble* or *water-soluble.* While water-soluble vitamins must be obtained each day from the foods we eat, a greater amount of fat-soluble vitamins can be stored in our bodies. Fat-soluble vitamins include vitamins A, D, E, and K; all other vitamins are water-soluble. The B vitamins are water-soluble. In addition, some vitamins are easily destroyed by light or heat; others are stable.

- *Functions:* Each vitamin plays a unique role in maintaining the health and well-being of you and your baby. Knowing the function of each will help you make sound food choices and understand the importance of the food recommendations.
- *Dangers from too little or too much:* You should know what current research shows about deficiencies and overdoses. Too little can cause a deficiency that retards growth and development. (Women in developing countries aren't the only ones who develop vitamin deficiencies.) Too much of some vitamins can be toxic, causing permanent damage to you or your baby.
- *Recommendations during pregnancy:* This is an estimate of the amount of the vitamin you should have in one day. Your dietary intake may be less than the RDA but still be adequate, since the recommendations are set at generous levels. This column also gives the amount needed during lactation.
- *Food sources:* These lists will help you choose food rich in particular vitamins. We encourage you to try some new ones. There may be some surprises on our lists.
- *Getting the maximum:* Vitamins are fragile! These tips will help you store, prepare, and cook foods so you get the most vitamins from them.

THE B VITAMINS: Thiamin

OTHER NAMES

B_1
Former names: vitamin F, antiberiberi factor

PHYSICAL CHARACTERISTICS

Water-soluble
Stable in heat when dry or in acid; destroyed in alkaline solutions (as when cooked with baking soda)
Destroyed when exposed to air
Nutlike or yeasty odor and flavor

FUNCTIONS

Promotes breakdown of carbohydrate to provide energy
Aids in digestion
Related to normal appetite
Essential for functioning of nervous system
Maintains muscle tone for heart function
Necessary for maternal and fetal growth
Carbohydrate is essential for fetal brain development, and thiamin is essential for carbohydrate to be used for this task
Thiamin must be supplied or brain development will be impaired

DANGERS FROM TOO LITTLE

Deficiency can cause depression or irritability, loss of appetite, fatigue, constipation, backache, insomnia, and cramps (all are symptoms common during pregnancy, however, and not necessarily caused by a thiamin deficiency)

Severe deficiency can result in beriberi, which is characterized by nausea, irritability, poor appetite, confusion, fatigue, muscle aches, and damage to the nervous system leading to paralysis
If maternal deficiency is severe, infant may be born with congenital beriberi
Deficiencies are most commonly associated with high alcohol consumption

DANGERS FROM TOO MUCH

There is no evidence of toxicity from thiamin (174)

RECOMMENDATIONS DURING PREGNANCY

RDA = 1.5 milligrams/day
For lactation: 1.6 milligrams/day

Thiamin needs depend on caloric intake because thiamin is needed to utilize the carbohydrate that provides calories
Generally, most pregnant women easily meet their needs for thiamin (172)

FOOD SOURCES

Lean pork (best source)
Liver
Legumes, peas, soybeans, kidney beans
Enriched or whole-grain breads and cereals (enriched grains have the thiamin lost in processing restored)
Nuts and seeds
Asparagus
Wheat germ
Lean meat
Fish
The best sources of thiamin are in meat, but vegetarians who

eat plenty of whole grains and enriched breads and cereals can get adequate thiamin

GETTING THE MAXIMUM

Do not wash rice before cooking it
Cook vegetables in as little water as possible
Do not add baking soda to water when cooking beans, greens, or any vegetable; it destroys the thiamin
Overcooking beef destroys thiamin
Using antacids for nausea reduces thiamin utilization; some diuretic medications increase urinary loss of thiamin
Absorption is reduced by consuming alcohol and sugar, and by drinking tea with meals
Sugar requires thiamin for its metabolism in cells, so indirectly increases thiamin needs

---

THE B VITAMINS: Niacin

OTHER NAMES

B_3
Nicotinic acid*
Nicotinamide†
Niacinamide

PHYSICAL CHARACTERISTICS

Water-soluble
One of the most stable of the B vitamins

FUNCTIONS

Needed for breakdown of glucose, protein, and fat to provide energy

Present in all body tissues and therefore very important to total growth and development of fetus
Promotes healthy skin, nerves, and digestive tract
Needed to convert folate acid to active form

DANGERS FROM TOO LITTLE

Effects of niacin deficiency in pregnant women have not been investigated
Deficiency (pellagra) marked by irritability, loss of appetite, swollen tongue, insomnia, skin rash, headache, and digestive disorders

DANGERS FROM TOO MUCH

No known toxic effects, but huge doses of nicotinic acid can cause flushing, itching, and gastrointestinal problems and can be dangerous to diabetics

RECOMMENDATIONS DURING PREGNANCY

RDA = 17 milligrams niacin equivalents†/day
For lactation: 20 milligrams niacin equivalents†/day

Pregnant women seem to have increased ability to form niacin from tryptophan (189) due to increased estrogen levels (198)

FOOD SOURCES

Complete proteins: liver, lean meat, poultry, fish, shellfish, eggs
Whole and enriched grains, bran cereals
Legumes, pinto beans, peas, peanut butter, peanuts
Tomatoes
Spinach
Potatoes
Milk

GETTING THE MAXIMUM

Use as little water as possible in cooking
Do not completely thaw frozen fish before cooking. Niacin is lost if liquid from fish is discarded
Alcoholic consumption contributes to niacin deficiency
Diets high in corn and cornmeal can contribute to deficiency
Niacin deficiency is uncommon in people who eat complete and adequate protein, especially from meat and milk

* Not the same as nicotine in cigarettes

† Niacin can be converted from tryptophan, an amino acid that is present in all complete proteins. Niacin equivalents (NEs) equal the amount of niacin itself plus the amount formed from the tryptophan.

THE B VITAMINS: Riboflavin

OTHER NAMES

B_2
Former name: vitamin G

PHYSICAL CHARACTERISTICS

Water-soluble
Yellow-green fluorescent color
Relatively heat stable; stable in oxygen; destroyed by light and alkali (baking soda)

FUNCTIONS

Essential for breakdown from carbohydrate, fat, and protein to provide energy

Necessary for growth and building tissue
Promotes good vision and healthy skin
Necessary for conversion of tryptophan to niacin and B_6, and folate to active forms

DANGERS FROM TOO LITTLE

Lack of riboflavin was once thought to cause prematurity, but recent studies show no association
Symptoms of deficiency include cracked and sore mouth, watery bloodshot eyes, swollen tongue, and dermatitis

DANGERS FROM TOO MUCH

No known danger from excesses (172; 174)

RECOMMENDATIONS DURING PREGNANCY

RDA = 1.6 milligrams/day
For lactation: first 6 months, 1.8 milligrams/day; second 6 months, 1.7 milligrams/day

Strict vegetarians may have difficulty meeting their riboflavin needs
Most pregnant women easily meet their needs for riboflavin

FOOD SOURCES

About half of riboflavin comes from dairy products; a quarter comes from meat
Vegetarians who don't eat any foods from animal sources should eat more green leafy vegetables, whole grains, dried peas, beans, nuts, and seeds to get enough riboflavin

Milk
Yogurt

Cheese, cottage cheese
Organ meats, liver (including chicken livers)
Lean meat
Leafy green vegetables (especially spinach, asparagus, broccoli, and greens)
Whole grains, barley
Enriched breads, cereals (enriched grains have the riboflavin lost in processing restored)
Dried peas and beans
Nuts and seeds
Eggs

GETTING THE MAXIMUM

Store milk away from light in an opaque container—milk exposed to sunlight for several hours can lose half its riboflavin
Do not add baking soda to water when cooking greens or vegetables
Certain diuretics and antibiotics can increase urinary excretion of riboflavin

---

THE B VITAMINS: Vitamin B_6

OTHER NAMES

Pyridoxine
Pyridoxal
PLP (Pyridoxal phosphate)
Pyridoxamine

PHYSICAL CHARACTERISTICS

Water-soluble
Generally stable; can be destroyed by light and heat

FUNCTIONS

Helps to absorb protein and fat
Helps energy production
Especially important for development of fetal brain and nerve tissue
Necessary for conversion of tryptophan to niacin
Affects hormones related to stress
Associated with immunity to disease and production of red blood cells

DANGERS FROM TOO LITTLE

Symptoms of deficiency are anemia, nervousness, dry mouth, weakness, dermatitis, nausea, and tingling sensation in fingers and toes (all are symptoms common during pregnancy, however, and are not necessarily caused by a B_6 deficiency)
Babies born to mothers with poor B_6 status tend to have lower scores on APGAR tests for responses given immediately after birth than those born to mothers with good B_6 status (160)

DANGERS FROM TOO MUCH

Toxicity resulting in neurological damage has been seen in women taking large doses of B_6 for treatment of premenstrual syndrome over a prolonged time (42)

RECOMMENDATIONS DURING PREGNANCY

RDA = 2.2 milligrams/day
For lactation: 2.1 milligrams/day

Need is related to protein intake
Needs increase during pregnancy because of high fetal demand for B_6

Women who took the pill until just prior to pregnancy sometimes have difficulty absorbing vitamin B_6, thus increasing their need, but newer low-dose oral contraceptives may not have this effect

Evidence exists that B_6 is used more efficiently during pregnancy due to hormonal changes (197)

Some researchers have found B_6 can reduce poor appetite, depression (90), and morning sickness (190); other studies show no evidence that B_6 is effective in treating nausea (109)

FOOD SOURCES

Widely distributed in unprocessed foods

Wheat germ
Meat, especially liver and kidney
Whole-grain cereals, bread
Bananas
Beans, peas, soybeans
Nuts and seeds
Corn
Pork
Poultry
Fish, especially smelt
Oatmeal
Vegetables, especially green leafy vegetables
Avocado
Cauliflower
Cabbage
Bran
Yams

GETTING THE MAXIMUM

Eat whole-grain cereals and breads; up to 90% of B_6 is destroyed by processing and is not replaced by enrichment (174)

B_6 from vegetable sources is more resistant to losses than B_6 from animal sources; include fresh vegetables in your daily diet

About 40 medications, including those used to treat tuberculosis, interfere with B_6 utilization

From 15% to 70% of B_6 can be lost in freezing fruits and vegetables (174)—fresh is best for B_6

THE B VITAMINS: Vitamin B_{12}

OTHER NAMES

Cobalamin

Extrinsic factor (called "extrinsic" because it cannot be made by the body)

PHYSICAL CHARACTERISTICS

Water-soluble

Fairly stable but can be destroyed by heat

Red-colored

Only vitamin known to contain the mineral cobalt

FUNCTIONS

Necessary for formation of proteins

Essential for cell division and growth; especially important for development and function of brain and nerve cells

Important for red blood-cell formation; releases folate for use by tissues

DANGERS FROM TOO LITTLE

Chronic deficiency (pernicious anemia) can cause permanent damage to the nervous system, but this condition is rare except among those with abnormal gastrointestinal functioning, strict vegetarians, alcoholics, and some people receiving certain medications

Deficiencies develop very slowly, usually over several years

B_{12} needs secretions from the stomach wall to be absorbed; malfunction of this mechanism rather than a lack of B_{12} in your diet is more likely to be the cause of a deficiency—your doctor is responsible for detecting this problem

Long-term antibiotic treatment can lead to B_{12} deficiency

Deficiency of B_{12} also yields folate deficiency since B_{12} is needed for folate use

A few infants born to strict vegetarians have vitamin B_{12} deficiency in the first 6 months of life (166)

DANGERS FROM TOO MUCH

B_{12} has no known toxicity to adults, but there have been no studies on its fetal effects (111)

RECOMMENDATIONS DURING PREGNANCY

RDA = 2.2 micrograms/day

For lactation: 2.6 micrograms/day

Though most water-soluble vitamins are excreted in urine if taken in excess, B_{12} is bound to a protein and stored in the liver—the fetus can draw on these reserves

B_{12} supplements at RDA levels are recommended for strict vegetarians (172; 174)
Vegetarians who eat eggs, milk, and cheese can get enough B_{12} from these foods (95)

FOOD SOURCES

Found almost exclusively in animal foods

Liver, kidney, lean meats
Fish
Oysters, clams, crabmeat
Cheese (especially cottage cheese)
Egg yolk

Some found in fermented foods: sauerkraut, tofu (soybean curd)

GETTING THE MAXIMUM

More B_{12} is absorbed during pregnancy
Boiling milk for long periods of time will reduce B_{12}
Factors that decrease absorption of B_{12} include lack of secretions in stomach and gastrointestinal problems

---

THE B VITAMINS: Folate

OTHER NAMES

Folacin
Folic acid
Pteroylglutamic acid (PGA)
Former names: vitamin M, citrovorum factor

PHYSICAL CHARACTERISTICS

Water-soluble
Deteriorates at room temperature and in sunlight
Destroyed by high heat

FUNCTIONS

Folate is a critical vitamin during pregnancy (197) because needs are high and low blood levels are fairly common
Folate is necessary for cell division—the basis of growth of the fetus
Essential component of blood cells and enzymes
Important for increasing number of blood cells
Necessary for utilization of some amino acids

DANGERS FROM TOO LITTLE

Deficiency can cause megaloblastic anemia in the mother

DANGERS FROM TOO MUCH

There are no reports of toxicity due to excess
Some studies report low maternal folate levels are associated with increases in congenital malformations, low-birth-weight babies, and third-trimester bleeding (202)

RECOMMENDATIONS DURING PREGNANCY

RDA = 400 micrograms/day
For lactation: first 6 months, 280 micrograms/day; second 6 months, 260 micrograms/day

The 400-microgram level during pregnancy can be met by a good diet without fortification or supplementation (174)

Taking folate supplements is controversial: The RDA subcommittee recommends more research and increased fruit and vegetable consumption, but does not recommend routine folate supplements at this time; others advocate folate supplements for all pregnant women (197)

Large amounts of folate are not given because they can mask detection of pernicious anemia; for this reason, the Food and Drug Administration has set limits on the amount of folate, per tablet, that can be sold without a doctor's prescription

Prenatal vitamin supplements have more folate than regular multivitamins

Pregnant teens, women carrying more than one fetus, and women who are in high-risk groups may be advised to take folate supplements (172)

FOOD SOURCES

Leafy green vegetables (spinach, greens, romaine lettuce)
Liver, kidney, liver sausage
Legumes: garbanzos, kidney beans, lima beans
Asparagus
Broccoli
Avocado
Brussels sprouts
Orange juice
Pineapple juice
Potatoes
Egg yolk
Melons
Strawberries
Nuts and seeds

GETTING THE MAXIMUM

Folate is stable in orange juice because it is protected by vitamin C
Eat fruits and vegetables raw for maximum benefit
Folate is lost whenever high temperature or large amounts of water are used in cooking
Refrigerate fruits and vegetables to prevent loss of the folate
Chronic alcoholics cannot absorb the common dietary forms of folate; the synthetic form of the vitamin is better utilized
More folate is destroyed by microwave cooking than by other cooking methods
Certain medications (anticonvulsants), alcohol, and cigarettes may interfere with folate utilization

THE B VITAMINS: Pantothenic Acid

OTHER NAMES

None

PHYSICAL CHARACTERISTICS

Water-soluble
Can be destroyed by alkali, acid, or heat

FUNCTIONS

Essential for metabolism of carbohydrate and protein from foods into substances that can be used in the human body
Necessary to make hormones
Necessary for formation of pigment in hemoglobin (makes red blood red)

Pantothenic acid will *not* prevent hair from turning gray

DANGERS FROM TOO LITTLE

Severe deficiencies are infrequent in humans except for those under extreme physical stress, but low intake can lower resistance to infection and increase irritability, cramps, fatigue, depression, and burning feeling in feet

DANGERS FROM TOO MUCH

No known toxicity (172)
Excess may cause diarrhea (63)

RECOMMENDATIONS DURING PREGNANCY

No specific RDA has been established for pregnant or nonpregnant women
An adequate level is estimated to be 4 to 7 milligrams/day for adults
Supplements are not necessary because foods provide a ready source
Some pantothenic acid is made in the digestive tract

FOOD SOURCES

Pantothenic acid is found in all living matter

Beef liver, kidney
Milk
Fish, especially trout
Poultry
Whole grains
Legumes, peas
Egg yolk
Most vegetables, especially mushrooms and potatoes

GETTING THE MAXIMUM

Less processed foods are richest in pantothenic acid
Canning destroys 50% to 62% of the vitamin in fruits and vegetables
Choose fresh fruits and vegetables as well as whole-grain cereals and breads—40% of wheat's pantothenic acid is lost in processing

---

THE B VITAMINS: Biotin

OTHER NAMES

Former names: vitamin H, co-enzyme R

PHYSICAL CHARACTERISTICS

Water-soluble
Sulfur containing
Stable in heat, acid
Readily destroyed by air and light

FUNCTIONS

Necessary for release of energy from other nutrients
Necessary for synthesis of some fats

DANGERS FROM TOO LITTLE

Deficiency in humans causes specific types of skin problems, loss of appetite, muscle pain, nausea, and hair loss

DANGERS FROM TOO MUCH

There are no known risks from excesses, but no specific toxicity studies have been conducted during pregnancy (172)

RECOMMENDATIONS DURING PREGNANCY

No specific values for pregnancy or lactation
30 to 100 micrograms/day estimated to be adequate for adults

Most diets contain 150 to 300 micrograms of biotin daily—enough to meet the needs of pregnancy
Some biotin is made in the digestive tract

FOOD SOURCES

Biotin is present in most foods

Egg yolk
Liver, kidney
Meat
Tomatoes
Cauliflower
Mushrooms
Dried peas and beans, soybeans
Nuts

GETTING THE MAXIMUM

Biotin is destroyed by raw egg whites, but it would take a diet of 25 to 30 raw egg whites a day to cause any problem; cooking egg whites renders biotin blockers harmless
Some biotin may be lost in cooking water—the less water you use in cooking, the better

Some biotin is synthesized by bacteria in the intestine; taking antibiotics reduces this production

VITAMIN A

OTHER NAMES

Anti-infective vitamin
Animal form: retinol
Vegetable form: carotene, especially beta carotene

PHYSICAL CHARACTERISTICS

Fat-soluble
Can be protected by antioxidants (vitamins C and E)
Fairly stable but can be destroyed by high temperature, air, sunlight, and drying

FUNCTIONS

Maintains epithelial tissue (internal and external "skin")—over $\frac{1}{4}$ acre in the average adult
Required for growth, cell differentiation, and development of fetus
Increases resistance to infection
Promotes bone and tooth development
Necessary for vision in dim light
Related to hormone production

DANGERS OF TOO LITTLE

Symptoms of deficiency include loss of appetite, poor growth, infections, eye changes that cause night blindness, eye disease, and blindness

Prenatal vitamin A deficiency has been related to eye abnormalities and impaired vision in children (93)

DANGERS FROM TOO MUCH

The symptoms of excessive vitamin A intake are headache, vomiting, drying of mucous membranes, bone abnormalities, and liver damage

Toxic doses can be obtained only by supplements or concentrates such as fish oil, not by eating too many vegetables

There is a high incidence of spontaneous abortion and birth defects in babies born to mothers who took large doses of vitamin A during the first trimester of pregnancy (174)

Women taking Accutane or other drugs for acne that contain vitamin A should take measures to avoid conception during treatment (105)

Large amounts of retinol can be toxic to the mother

Carotene is not known to be toxic, but excesses of carotene may cause skin to discolor

RECOMMENDATIONS DURING PREGNANCY

RDA = 800 retinol equivalents*(RE)/day (the same amount as for nonpregnant females)

For lactation: first 6 months, 1300 RE/day; after 6 months, 1200 RE/day (to replace losses in milk)

Fish liver oil, previously used as a vitamin A supplement, is no longer recommended

FOOD SOURCES

Liver (outstanding source because that's where vitamin A is stored in animals), liver sausage

* Each RE is equal to 1 microgram of retinol or 6 micrograms of carotene. Carotene is absorbed less effectively than retinol and must be converted to active retinol in the body to be used.

Milk
Cheese
Fortified margarine
Butter

Color—yellow, green, and orange—is a clue in choosing foods rich in carotene

Dark-green leafy vegetables: spinach, broccoli, greens (*not* iceberg lettuce or celery)

Deep-yellow or orange vegetables and fruits: carrots, winter squash, apricots, pumpkins, cantaloupe, sweet potato, papaya, tomatoes

GETTING THE MAXIMUM

The potency of vitamin A is protected when antioxidants such as vitamins C and E are present or added

Absorption is enhanced by presence of fat, protein, and vitamin E

Vitamin A is contained in fat and lost when fat is removed from lowfat or skim milk; if you choose nonfat milk or yogurt, be sure it is *fortified* with vitamin A

Mineral oil interferes with absorption of vitamin A—do not use mineral oil as a laxative or use low-calorie salad dressings containing mineral oil

Tannic acid from tea can impair vitamin A absorption

VITAMIN C

OTHER NAMES

Ascorbic acid

PHYSICAL CHARACTERISTICS

Water-soluble
The least stable of vitamins; destroyed by air when in liquids; destroyed by heat
Destruction accelerated by light and by exposure to some metals

FUNCTIONS

Necessary for normal functioning of all cells
Essential for development of bones, teeth, and blood vessels
Necessary for the formation of the protein collagen, which holds skin and bones together—sometimes called "cell cement"
Greatly increases absorption of iron from plant foods—important during pregnancy because iron is needed for the increased blood volume
Converts inactive form of folate to active form needed for blood cells
Essential for metabolism of some amino acids and hormones
There is no proof that vitamin C helps to prevent illness such as colds, but it is important in the healing process and it is a natural antihistamine. While vitamin C won't prevent a cold, it reduces symptoms if you have one
Vitamin C may be added to foods as a preservative to prevent oxidation (turning brown)

DANGERS FROM TOO LITTLE

Symptoms of mild deficiency are bleeding gums, easy bruising, slow healing, weakness, aches, and bone pain

Severe deficiency is called scurvy

Very low maternal intake is associated with increased rates of premature birth (193)

DANGERS FROM TOO MUCH

Symptoms of excessive intake are diarrhea, rashes, and frequent urination

High intake can cause kidney stones and gout in some individuals

Megadoses of vitamin C during pregnancy can condition the child to greater need *after* birth; a newborn of a mother who takes excessive vitamin C may experience temporary but painful deficiency until the baby adjusts to more normal levels (called "rebound" or "conditioned" scurvy) (202)

Individuals who take excess vitamin C in concentrated pill form can condition their body to needing more vitamin C, thus causing symptoms of deficiency (bleeding gums) when they stop taking the pills

RECOMMENDATIONS DURING PREGNANCY

RDAs are increased from 60 to 70 milligrams/day during pregnancy to meet the demands for fetal growth and maternal tissues

For lactation: first 6 months, 95 milligrams/day; second 6 months, 90 milligrams/day

Vitamin C is needed each day

Most Americans get more than enough Vitamin C

Women who smoke cigarettes or take aspirin regularly have an increased need for vitamin C which can be met by drinking one 4 oz. glass of orange juice (50 milligrams of vitamin C) each day or taking a 50-milligram supplement if increased consumption of fruits and vegetables is not possible

FOOD SOURCES

Citrus fruits, juices
Acerola cherries
Green peppers
Strawberries
Tomatoes, tomato juice
Brussels sprouts
Melons, cantaloupe
Mangos, papaya
Kiwi
Broccoli
Cabbage
Pineapple
Cauliflower
Spinach, kale
Potatoes
Mustard, collard greens

GETTING THE MAXIMUM

Store foods in a cool, dark place
Do not cut or peel fruits and vegetables until ready to serve; bake potatoes whole
Store juices in covered containers
Cook vegetables quickly or steam them
Dried fruits have practically no vitamin C
Cooking foods in copper pots reduces vitamin C value

VITAMIN D

OTHER NAMES

Calciferol
Several forms: ergocalciferol (D_2), cholecalciferol (D_3), irradiated ergosterol,* 7-dehydrocholesterol

PHYSICAL CHARACTERISTICS

Fat-soluble
Generally stable

FUNCTIONS

Essential for baby's development and mother's maintenance of cell structures
Necessary for maintenance of normal levels of calcium and phosphorus in blood

DANGERS FROM TOO LITTLE

Low levels of vitamin D may predispose a woman to soft bones that affect posture and cause lower-back pain
Severe deficiency is rickets, characterized by bone deformities
Maternal deficiency has been associated with seizures and rickets of newborns (46)

DANGERS FROM TOO MUCH

Overdoses can occur with as little as five times daily need
Toxicity symptoms include calcium deposits in soft tissues (especially in kidneys), headache, diarrhea, and nausea

* *Irradiated* means that the vitamin D was activated by exposure to light. Don't be concerned about radiation.

In Gottingen, Germany, when huge doses of vitamin D were given to prevent rickets, babies were born with heart and facial defects and mental retardation (67)

RECOMMENDATIONS DURING PREGNANCY

RDA for pregnancy *and* lactation = 10 micrograms/day (400 IU vitamin D)

Women who have had multiple pregnancies in a short period of time or who have breast-fed for long periods just prior to this pregnancy may have depleted vitamin D stores

Breast-fed infants need supplementary vitamin D or exposure to sunlight; infant formulas are fortified with vitamin D (46)

FOOD SOURCES

Vitamin D-fortified milk (approximately 98% of milk sold in the United States is fortified with vitamin D)

Fortified margarine

Liver

Canned salmon, sardines, herring

Egg yolk

Cereals fortified with vitamin D

GETTING THE MAXIMUM

Vitamin D is formed in the skin when it is exposed to light; also produced when ergosterol from plants is exposed to light (the form of vitamin D added to fortified foods)

Drink vitamin A- and D-fortified milk

VITAMIN E

OTHER NAMES

Tocotrienols
Tocopherol forms: alpha-tocopherol, beta-tocopherol, delta-tocopherol, gamma-tocopherol

PHYSICAL CHARACTERISTICS

Fat-soluble
Stable in heat but not in air, freezing, or sunlight

FUNCTIONS

Antioxidant—protects vitamins A and C and polyunsaturated fats in the body from destruction by oxygen
Helps form normal blood cells, muscle cells, and other tissues
There have been many claims for vitamin E: It is known as the antisterility vitamin, but affects only rat, not human, fertility
The relationship of vitamin E to a variety of other reproductive problems has not been documented for humans
Effectiveness in preventing permanent stretch marks has not been scientifically established

DANGERS FROM TOO LITTLE

Deficiency has not been seen in adults except those unable to absorb fats

DANGERS FROM TOO MUCH

Toxicity has not been documented in humans

RECOMMENDATIONS DURING PREGNANCY

RDA = 10 milligrams/day, based on alpha-tocopherol equivalents (alpha TE)
For lactation: first 6 months, 12 milligrams/day alpha TE; second 6 months, 11 milligrams/day alpha TE

The body has a great reserve of vitamin E in fatty tissues
There are no known benefits of supplementation in normal women; thus, supplements are not recommended (174)
Little vitamin E crosses the placenta until late in pregnancy, so premature infants have a low supply; premature infants often receive supplements of vitamin E
Deficiencies are seen in very-low-birth-weight infants (197);
The need for vitamin E increases in relation to increased consumption of polyunsaturated fats. Fortunately, they are usually together in foods, such as margarine

FOOD SOURCES

Vegetable oils (especially soybean, corn, sunflower oils)
Whole grains (especially wheat germ)
Green leafy vegetables
Mayonnaise
Seeds and nuts, sunflower seeds
Brown rice
Avocado
Margarine

GETTING THE MAXIMUM

Needs increase as polyunsaturated fat sources increase, but these same foods supply this vitamin
Normal bile secretion and pancreatic function are necessary for absorption

Mineral oil used as laxative removes vitamin E from the body (this laxative is discouraged at all times, but particularly during pregnancy)

VITAMIN K

OTHER NAMES

Phylloquinone
Menaquinones
Menadione (a synthetic vitamin K)
Former name: antihemorrhagic vitamin

PHYSICAL CHARACTERISTICS

Fat-soluble
Synthetic form is water-soluble
Heat stable
Destroyed by light and strong acids

FUNCTIONS

Aids in blood clotting
Helps form some proteins found in bone, kidney, and tissues (174)
Some vitamin K is formed by intestinal synthesis
Vitamin K is given to newborns to prevent bleeding before their intestinal tract is ready to produce vitamin K

DANGERS FROM TOO LITTLE

Deficiency of vitamin K is unlikely except in newborn infants who cannot synthesize it or adults unable to absorb fats

DANGERS FROM TOO MUCH

Excesses may cause birth defects if taken in toxic dosage (93)
May be given by doctor during last few weeks of pregnancy or during labor to prevent hemorrhaging; levels should be carefully controlled to prevent adverse reactions

RECOMMENDATIONS DURING PREGNANCY

RDA for pregnancy *and* lactation = 65 micrograms/day

Vitamin K is readily available in commonly eaten foods and is produced in the body by intestinal bacteria
Mothers who are being treated with antibiotics may need supplements, because antibiotics reduce ability of gastrointestinal tract to produce vitamin K
Chronic diarrhea or poor absorption may increase need

FOOD SOURCES

Best sources: dark-green leafy vegetables, cabbage, and broccoli
Liver
Egg yolks
Lentils
Cauliflower
Milk

GETTING THE MAXIMUM

Store foods in a dark place, such as a refrigerator
Stable; no losses in cooking
Aspirin interferes with utilization of vitamin K (177)

6

Minerals: The Strong Supports

QUICK QUIZ

How much do you know about minerals? The correct answers are on page 293.

FILL IN THE BLANKS

1. ________________ is added to milk to increase calcium absorption.
2. ________________ is the only routinely recommended mineral supplement for normal, healthy pregnant women.
3. People whose municipal drinking water has added ____________ have fewer dental caries and have stronger bones.
4. Eating ice cubes may be an indication that you are deficient in ________________.
5. Everyone knows that salt contains sodium, but it contains even more ________________.

TRUE OR FALSE

___ 6. During pregnancy women should reduce their salt intake.

___ 7. Drinking tea inhibits the iron absorption from foods eaten at the same meal.

___ 8. Women who are over 30 years old need more calcium during pregnancy than do younger women.
___ 9. Shellfish, particularly oysters, are rich in zinc.
___ 10. Lowfat milk has less calcium than whole milk.

When you build a home, you want its supports to be strong and durable. In the human body, minerals determine the strength and durability of the structural support system.

Most of the "mineral deposits" in our bodies are in bones and teeth, which survive after the rest of the body is long gone. Sugar and spice may be very nice, but *minerals* are what boys and girls are really made of!

Minerals are strong and durable, in part because most of them are elements. An *element* consists of a single kind of atom that cannot be chemically broken into parts. Some minerals such as fluorine are used in the human body in a compound form (fluoride). We refer to these as minerals for simplicity.

Minerals used by the human body must be provided by diet—they cannot be manufactured internally. But some can be recycled and reused within the body. They have two functions: building and regulating. As builders, minerals help form the skeleton and soft tissues, and they form parts of vital body chemicals—such as iron in the hemoglobin of red blood cells and iodine in the thyroid hormone *thyroxine.* As regulators, minerals influence a wide variety of functions such as heartbeat, blood clotting, maintenance of body fluid pressure, nerve behavior, and transport of oxygen from lungs to tissues.

Here's a simplified explanation of how minerals build and

regulate. Electrically charged minerals, called *ions,* regulate body systems. Like magnets, some ions have minus charges; others have plus charges. The balance of plus- and minus-charged ions keeps fluid outside of cells from putting too much pressure on cell walls and maintains enough pressure inside cells to keep them from collapsing.

Some minerals are found in significant quantities in the body. These *macrominerals* are calcium, phosphorus, sodium, chlorine, potassium, magnesium, and sulfur. Others, equally essential though present in extremely small quantities, are called *microminerals* or, more commonly, *trace minerals.* The trace minerals include iron, chromium, cobalt, copper, fluorine, iodine, vanadium, manganese, molybdenum, nickel, selenium, silicon, tin, and zinc. Other minerals occur in nature but are not needed by the human body. Some, such as lead, cadmium, and mercury, are harmful or fatal if consumed in large amounts.

CALCIUM AND PHOSPHORUS

Calcium and phosphorus, which exist in a constant ratio in the blood, are team players in the body-building process, so we will discuss them together. During pregnancy and lactation, twelve hundred milligrams of each are recommended each day.

About 99 percent of the body's calcium and 80 percent of its phosphorus are found in bones and teeth. While we think of bones as durable and permanent, they actually are constantly being broken down and rebuilt. During the growing years, there's more building and rebuilding than breaking down. After about age twenty-five, there's much less growth in bones, although they continue breaking down. After menopause, bone loss is significantly greater than bone growth.

Calcium balance is regulated by hormones and involves vitamin D. Here's how it works. When blood calcium levels fall, the parathyroid gland secretes one of these hormones known as parathyroid hormone (PTH). PTH does two things: First, it triggers a release of calcium from bone. Second, it stimulates the kidney to produce an active form of vitamin D that has been supplied either from food or from sunlight. Vitamin D increases calcium absorption. The net result is normalized blood calcium levels.

Ultraviolet sunlight, absorbed through the skin, converts vitamin D's precursor, 7-dehydrocholesterol, into vitamin D. Women who live in northern climates, who work indoors, or who always wear clothing that shields them from sunlight may not absorb much of the precursor vitamin. Some studies show that vitamin D synthesis is slower on dark-pigmented skin (32). Because exposure to sunlight is so variable, you're better off drinking vitamin D–fortified milk. It provides both calcium and vitamin D to help absorb it. Women who neither have exposure to the sun nor drink milk may need vitamin D supplements, but only under medical supervision.

Pregnancy: A Calcium Countdown

During pregnancy, the placenta produces hormones (estrogen and human chorionic somatomammotropin) that simultaneously stimulate release of calcium *from* your bones and increase absorption and deposition of calcium *into* your bones. These hormones do not pass into the fetal bloodstream.

A placental form of vitamin D makes sure that calcium moves from you to baby. As your calcium blood level falls, the parathyroid gland pumps out PTH to trigger release of calcium from your bones. This demand, in conjunction with the action of prenatal hormones, requires a steady supply of calcium and, to some extent, vitamin D. If your diet doesn't provide enough calcium, it will be drawn from your bones to bring the blood level back to normal. Maintaining blood levels of calcium is essential because calcium regulates essential functions like muscle contractions and heartbeat rhythm. If the dietary supply is adequate, bone reserves will be either untouched or replaced (197). If calcium intake is low, particularly after several or closely spaced pregnancies, your bones can be weakened. Weak bones put a woman more at risk of osteoporosis later in life.

The fetus produces hormones of its own that promote deposits of calcium into bones. As the months progress, more and more calcium is deposited. By the third trimester, about three hundred milligrams a day, most of the RDA increase for pregnancy, is going to the baby. As fetal needs increase, maternal absorption of dietary calcium increases. One study showed that nonpregnant women absorbed 27 percent of dietary calcium; women five to six months pregnant absorbed 54 percent, and women at term absorbed 42 percent (by then the baby is about "built") (80).

Daily Double: Milk and Sunshine

Since many American women do not get enough calcium when not pregnant, it may take some dietary changes for a mother-to-be to meet her baby's needs for calcium and vitamin D as well as her own. While serious defects as the result of low dietary calcium intake are not widely documented, there is concern about the impact on the baby's bone calcification. A little calcium deficiency in the bones of a 7-pound baby is more significant than it is in a 125-pound woman (197).

Some people will tell you that the extraordinary demand for calcium during pregnancy causes tooth decay because calcium is drawn from your teeth, but no studies have confirmed this. Calcium reserves are in bones, not in teeth. The slight increase in cavities during pregnancy may be due to a change in the composition of the saliva in the mouth. This potential problem can be handled by brushing your teeth more often.

A total of twelve hundred milligrams of calcium a day is generally recommended for a healthy pregnant woman carrying one baby. Dr. Roy Pitkin points out that since it is nearly impossible to meet calcium requirements without dairy products, milk is "practically essential for the pregnant woman. The allowance for pregnancy—twelve hundred milligrams—is precisely that contained in one quart of milk. Individuals who do not consume milk or milk products will require calcium supplementation" (141).

It does not matter whether you eat yogurt or drink whole milk, skim milk, reconstituted dry milk, buttermilk, or carbonated milk—the calcium is still there and these foods are traditionally fortified with vitamin D, which boosts calcium absorption and utilization. Butter and cream, however, are *not* good sources of calcium. And you don't have to drink your milk from a glass, either. You can put it into pancakes, soups, casseroles, or puddings. You can have yogurt plain or fruited, frozen or as a flavored ready-to-drink liquid from the dairy case.

Milk also contains lactose, a carbohydrate that increases calcium absorption. Some women, unable to digest lactose, get diarrhea if they drink milk. Fermented dairy products, such as buttermilk, yogurt, and natural cheeses, contain less lactose and may be substituted for milk. Lactose-hydrolyzed milk, such as Lactaid, or drops that will "digest" the lactose in regular milk work well. The enzyme that breaks down lactose, called lactase, is available in pill form and should be taken with meals. Women who are lactose-intolerant are often able to drink milk in small quantities (172).

The following chart identifies food sources of calcium that are equivalent to one cup of milk. If you eat canned fish, consume the soft edible bones that contain the calcium. Canned tuna, shrimp, and boneless fish filets have little calcium. Although data are not available to include in our chart, we also recommend small smelt with edible bones, soft-shell crab, and the tips of ribs, chicken legs, and wings as unusually good calcium sources.

Foods containing oxalates (tea, green leafy vegetables, cola beverages, chocolate, and peanut butter) and high-fiber foods cut down the rate of calcium absorption. So, many high-calcium foods (spinach, rhubarb, baked beans) provide calcium that may not be well absorbed (132).

As you review the Calcium Sources table you may realize that some portions are huge—you aren't expected to eat two cups of cottage cheese or a cup of almonds. The point here is that this is how much of that food it would take to obtain the three hundred milligrams of calcium in one cup of milk. Look at the calorie counts, too—to meet your daily calcium need with ice cream would cost you 1880 calories!

GOOD CALCIUM SOURCES

RDA in pregnancy: 1200 milligrams per day
RDA in lactation: 1200 milligrams per day

FOODS	AMOUNT EQUAL OF CALCIUM* (ABOUT 300 MG)	CALORIES
Almonds	3/4 cup	607
Blackstrap molasses	2 tbsp.	85
Bok choy (Chinese cabbage), cooked	2 cups	40
Broccoli, cooked	2 cups	200
Cheddar cheese	1 1/2 oz.	170
Collard greens, frozen, chopped, cooked	1 cup	60
Cottage cheese, creamed	2 cups	400
Cottage cheese, lowfat 1%	1 3/4 cups	242
Custard, baked	1 cup	305
Fudgesicle	2	182
Ham and cheese sandwich	1	350
Ice cream, regular vanilla (10% fat)	1 3/4 cups	470
Ice cream, rich vanilla (16% fat)	2 cups	700
Kale, cooked	1 3/4 cups	65
Kefir	1 cup	160
Mackerel, canned (Jack-type only)	3/4 cup	225
Milk, lowfat 1%	8 oz.	102
Milk, lowfat 2%	8 oz.	120
Milk, skim	8 oz.	86
Milk, whole	8 oz.	157
Milk, whole goat	8 oz.	168
Mozzarella cheese (part-skim)	2 oz.	140

FOODS	AMOUNT EQUAL OF CALCIUM* (ABOUT 300 MG)	CALORIES
Orange, grapefruit or apple juice, calcium-fortified	8 oz.	110
Parmesan cheese, grated	4 tbsp. ($\frac{3}{4}$ oz.)	100
Pizza, cheese, thin crust	2 pieces	306
Potatoes, au gratin	1 cup	322
Processed cheese, American	$1\frac{3}{4}$ oz.	186
Processed cheese, American sliced, reduced fat	$1\frac{1}{2}$ oz.	105
Rhubarb, cooked, sweetened†	1 cup	280
Ricotta cheese, part-skim	$\frac{1}{2}$ cup	170
Salmon, canned (with bones)	$4\frac{1}{2}$ oz.	200
Sardines, canned (with bones)	6–7 med.	160
Spinach, cooked†	$1\frac{1}{4}$ cups	60
Swiss or Gruyère cheese	1 oz.	115
Tofu, soybean curd, firm (processed with calcium sulfate)	$\frac{1}{2}$ cup	183
Tomato soup, prepared with milk	2 cups	320
Tostada (bean, chicken, or beef)	2	500
Turnip greens	$1\frac{1}{4}$ cups	70
Yogurt, drinkable (fruit or chocolate flavored)	1 cup	175
Yogurt, frozen	1 cup	220
Yogurt, plain, lowfat	1 cup	144
Yogurt, sweetened, lowfat, flavored	1 cup	240

* One cup of milk contains 300 mg of calcium.

† These foods contain substances which tend to block calcium's absorption. So while calcium is in the food, it may not be available to your body.

Calcium Supplements

If you don't drink milk because you do not like it, are lactose intolerant, or are a strict vegetarian, your doctor may prescribe calcium and vitamin D supplements. It's up to your doctor or a registered dietitian to decide whether or not you need calcium or vitamin D supplements.

Supplements made with calcium carbonate or calcium citrate, taken with or at the end of a meal, are absorbed best (79).

You can test absorbability by placing a calcium tablet in a little vinegar. Stir it every few minutes. It should break up (not dissolve) within 30 minutes. If it doesn't, choose a different product. A new form of calcium called CCM calcium, which is calcium bound to citric and malic acids, is being used to fortify orange and apple juice and grapefruit-juice cocktail. These two acids are typically found in citrus and apple juices. CCM calcium is particularly well absorbed because it is already dissolved and the citric acid and vitamin C in the juices also boost iron absorption (44). Calcium-fortified juices are a good way to increase both calcium and fruit consumption. They provide a nondairy option and a refreshing beverage for meals and snacks. We were surprised that we couldn't see or taste the calcium in the fruit juice.

Studies show that some hard, compressed calcium tablets manage to get through the digestive tract virtually undissolved. Do the vinegar test if you use tablets for extra calcium.

If you would rather take supplements than drink milk because you are concerned about the calories in milk, consider eliminating other less nutritious sources of calories first. If weight gain is a problem, choose skim milk and lowfat yogurt and cheese. Drinking milk is a simple, inexpensive way to meet a variety of nutrient needs, not only for calcium, phosphorus, and vitamin D, but for protein, riboflavin, and vitamin B_{12} as well. A milk-fed fetus is more likely to be a blue-ribbon baby than one who has to depend on less reliable sources of nutrients consumed by the mother.

Some studies suggest that calcium influences blood pressure, and that calcium supplements may be used to control pregnancy-induced hypertension (188). While the association warrants further research, the Subcommittee on Dietary Intake and Nutrient Supplements does not consider data firm enough at this time to recommend calcium supplements for prevention or treatment of pregnancy-induced hypertension.

SODIUM, CHLORIDE, AND POTASSIUM

Standard dietary advice suggests Americans cut back on salt. Typical intakes of salt (sodium chloride) are higher than most people need. As for sodium, the worrisome component of salt, an adult over the age of eighteen actually needs only five hundred milligrams per day. This minimum assumes normal body temperature without prolonged perspiration, which increases the need for sodium.

Studies show that typical consumption of sodium in the United States ranges from 4000 to 5800 milligrams daily. About one-third is sodium naturally found in food; another one-third is added during processing; the remaining one-third is added in cooking or at the table (66).

More sodium is needed during pregnancy and lactation than at any other time of life, but virtually all women meet this need with their normal intake of salt. Pregnant women are sometimes told to restrict salt to prevent weight gain, swelling, and pregnancy-induced hypertension (toxemia). But cutting back too severely can be harmful to both mother and baby. Here's why.

Salt is a combination of the minerals sodium and chloride. Sodium, a positive ion, and chloride, a negative ion (see page 162 for discussion of ions) are attracted to each other as dry substances and form a very durable bond. When they are put into a liquid, however, they separate and return to their ionic forms. In the body, salt exists as sodium and chloride ions in the bloodstream. Along with potassium, these minerals help regulate fluids in cells.

One principle behind fluid balance is that water "follows" sodium. If you have ever sprinkled salt on cucumbers, you have seen this mechanism at work. After a few minutes, the salt draws liquid out of the cucumbers. Sodium *outside* of body cells draws water out in a similar way. If it were not for potassium and chloride *inside* the cells, you would be left with cells that are as limp as salted cucumbers!

Some people seem very sensitive to salt. If they consume excessive amounts, their cell walls cannot hold back the water, which is drawn into the bloodstream. As the volume of fluid in the blood increases, blood pressure increases. This condition is known as *hypertension* or *high blood pressure.*

During pregnancy, however, the blood volume increases by about 50 percent for a single fetus, and even more in multiple pregnancies (202). As blood volume expands, the amount of water held in reserve in cells also expands. Sometimes, the cells get so full that they swell. This swelling is called *edema.* Some degree of edema is normal during pregnancy (see chapter 8). Some extra fluid is retained by changes in hormonal regulation systems in pregnancy.

The normal edema of pregnancy should not be treated by restricting salt or taking diuretics. Diuretics, often called water pills, are designed to eliminate water from the body. You need more fluid during pregnancy—for expanding blood and growing cells, and for maternal reserves that will play a role during delivery. The added fluid requires increased amounts of electrolytes such as sodium, potassium, and chloride. Ironically, swelling requires more, not less salt. Animal studies showed that when sodium was severely restricted during pregnancy, it inhibited the normal expansion of blood volume, thereby limiting the fetus's supply of nutrients. The result was smaller fetuses (197).

If swelling is excessive, there is usually a medical reason. Edema is a symptom of several serious problems and warrants examination by your doctor (see chapter 8). Women with diagnosed hypertension may need to restrict foods high in salt. If diuretics or medications are required, they will be used with very careful medical monitoring.

Current medical opinion holds that pregnant women should not limit salt and should salt food to taste. Most of us are aware of the high levels of sodium in some processed foods; in addition, sodium (and chloride) occurs naturally in foods. That business about pregnant women craving pickles may not be so crazy. Most pickles contain a lot of salt—and women need more salt during pregnancy. Pregnant women should have at least two thousand to three thousand milligrams of sodium per day (202). That amount can be obtained from a varied diet without any major effort to restrict or increase salt intake.

Like sodium and chloride, *potassium* helps regulate fluid balance and fluid volume in cells. It also is vital to the action of the heart, helps transmit nerve impulses, and helps maintain blood pressure. Unless you perspire profusely day after day, or unless you are taking a medication that causes potassium loss, you can get adequate potassium from foods. Potassium deficiencies are rare in this country, except as a result of vomiting, chronic diarrhea, protein malnutrition, or taking certain medications.

The average potassium consumption of adults depends largely on their eating habits. Those who eat plenty of fruits and vegetables get more potassium. On average, urban white adults eat about twenty-five hundred milligrams per day and black adults eat about one thousand milligrams daily (100). The estimated minimum potassium requirement for adults, set by the RDA, is two thousand milligrams. Many people get less; they should eat more fruits and vegetables and drink more milk. Doing just this will meet the potassium needs of pregnancy.

Megadoses of potassium supplements can cause imbalances leading to muscular paralysis, abnormal heartbeat rhythm, and even cardiac arrest (174). There is a reported case of a two-month-old infant who died from being given liquid potassium supplements to treat colic—a treatment suggested by the late Adelle Davis (40). While this is extreme, it is mentioned to illustrate the potential dangers of supplementing your own or your child's diet with vitamins and minerals as cures.

THE LAST (SULFUR) AND LEAST (MAGNESIUM) OF THE MACROMINERALS

Sulfur is a structural component of hair, skin, and nails. (If you have ever smelled burning hair, you've noticed the strange odor—that's sulfur dioxide.) Sulfur is a part of sev-

GOOD POTASSIUM SOURCES

No RDA for nonpregnant, pregnant or lactating adults
Recommendation based on requirements: 2000 to 3500 milligrams per day (174)

FOOD	PORTION	MILLIGRAM POTASSIUM	CALORIES
Potato, baked with skin	1, 7 oz.	844	220
Spaghetti with meat sauce	1 cup	665	330
Avocado	½	550	150
Cantaloupe	1 cup pieces	494	57
Oysters, simmered	3½ oz.	458	137
Broccoli, cooked	1 cup	456	44
Banana	1 med.	451	100
Yogurt, low-fat with fruit	1 cup	442	232
Milk, skim	1 cup	406	86
Milk, 2%	1 cup	377	120
Apricot halves	1 oz.	371	62
Scallops, breaded and fried	3½ oz.	333	215
Beef, lean sirloin	3 oz.	342	178
Fish, baked haddock	3 oz.	339	95
Prunes, dry	5	313	100
Grapes, seedless, green	1 cup	296	160
Ham, lean	3 oz.	269	133
Tomato	1 med.	254	24
English muffin, sourdough	1 med.	331	135
Pumpkin pie	1 slice	400	367
Chocolate milk, 1% fat	1 cup	425	160
Orange	1 med.	250	65
Turkey, roasted	3 oz.	250	145

FOOD	PORTION	MILLIGRAM POTASSIUM	CALORIES
Strawberries, fresh	1 cup	247	45
Chicken breast, roasted	½	240	193
Peanut butter	2 tbsp.	220	190
Cottage cheese, 2%	1 cup	217	205
Pear, Bartlett	1	208	98
Green pepper	½ cup chopped	98	12
Peas, canned	½ cup	92	92
Minestrone soup	1 cup	80	80
Grapefruit juice	6 oz.	75	70
Grapefruit juice	½ cup	200	45

eral amino acids and is found in the vitamins thiamin and biotin. If your diet contains adequate protein, you will receive sufficient sulfur during pregnancy. Eggs, meat, cheese, nuts, and legumes all have lots of sulfur.

Magnesium almost doesn't qualify as a macromineral because it is present in such small quantities. The RDA for magnesium during pregnancy is 320 milligrams. About 50 percent of magnesium in humans is stored in bones and teeth. It helps release energy from carbohydrate, fat, and protein, and maintains muscle contractability and nerve sensitivity.

Magnesium is a part of chlorophyll, the green pigment in plants. Green, leafy vegetables containing chlorophyll are excellent sources of magnesium. Other magnesium-containing foods are whole grains, bran, wheat germ, legumes, cocoa, nuts, soybeans, and whole grains. Since fiber reduces magnesium absorption, and many magnesium sources are fiber-rich, it is unclear how much magnesium is available to the body (161).

If your diet includes whole grains and vegetables, you will get enough magnesium. If, on the other hand, you suffer from prolonged diarrhea or vomiting, or use diuretics (not recommended during pregnancy), you may need to make a special effort to include magnesium-rich foods in your diet.

IRON

During pregnancy, iron is used for both fetal and maternal tissues, primarily to form red blood cells. As blood volume increases, so does the need for iron. Iron is part of the hemoglobin in these cells. It is the hemoglobin in red blood cells that carries oxygen to both maternal and fetal cells. If you reduce iron, you decrease the amount of hemoglobin and reduce the amount of oxygen, thereby limiting energy production. When you are pregnant, your baby's red blood cells get preferential treatment—you're the one who will be tired. Reduced hemoglobin and iron in the blood may also put stress on your heart because it must pump harder to supply oxygen to cells. This effort is intensified by the needs of the placenta and fetus.

Your need for iron changes over the nine months of pregnancy. During the first trimester, when you are still forming red blood cells at a fairly normal rate, demands are low and are satisfied by the iron saved when menstruation stops. During the second and third trimesters, the need for iron builds steadily. During the last months, the baby is most demanding as it builds it own iron reserves for the first three to four months after birth.

The baby takes what iron it needs, and doesn't pay a lot of attention to its mother's supplies or needs. Twins, who may not be able to gain ample iron stores, and premature babies, whose period of building iron reserves is shortened, may be iron-deficient during the first months after birth. Iron supplements are often prescribed for breast-fed twins and premies, and iron-supplemented formula is recommended for babies who are bottle-fed.

Having iron-deficiency anemia is hardly the best way for a woman to enter the demanding period of labor and delivery. An expanded blood volume allows for losses during delivery, but a large part of iron in red blood cells is retained after a vaginal delivery of a single baby and is returned to the mother's reserves as the blood volume returns to normal. Twice as much blood is lost during a cesarean delivery, postponing the mother's recovery of iron reserves (146).

Women in their childbearing years are more likely to be deficient in iron than in any other nutrient because iron reserves are tapped by monthly menstrual flow. Bleeding is the only significant way that iron is lost from the body. Women with heavy menstrual losses are more at risk for iron deficiencies than those who lose little blood. Menstruating women who take birth-control pills generally bleed only half as much as women who do not, and have significantly higher iron reserves as well (65).

Women who donate blood more than three times a year and those who take large amounts of aspirin (three-hundred-milligram tablets (four a day) are also at risk of iron deficiency (140; 165). Chronic use of aspirin can contribute to hemorrhaging, which depletes iron reserves.

Very few pregnant women are able to get enough iron from foods to meet the thirty milligrams RDA for the mineral.

Iron is present in foods in two forms: *heme iron,* found in meat, poultry, and fish, and *nonheme* iron, found in plant foods. Heme iron is absorbed far better than nonheme iron. Foods that contain phytates (whole grains), tannins (tea), and iron-binding polyphenols (coffee) further reduce nonheme iron absorption (97). On the other hand, you can boost absorption of iron by eating foods rich in heme iron or vitamin C at the same meal as nonheme foods. For example, the meat in a sandwich improves iron absorption from the bread; orange juice with cereal boosts the absorption from cereal; tomatoes boost absorption from spinach and other salad ingredients.

Although most of us eat far less heme than nonheme iron foods, we still get a much greater percentage of heme iron because it is better absorbed and is relatively unaffected by

---

You may have poor iron status if you

- Had heavy menstrual bleeding before pregnancy
- Eat little meat
- Eat few vegetables and fruits (vitamin C)
- Take large amounts of aspirin
- Give blood more than three times a year
- Are carrying more than one baby
- Are in your second or third trimester and do not take iron supplements (they are not prescribed or you do not take them regularly)
- Are in your teens and still growing
- Were pregnant with another baby less than two years ago (202)

---

other substances (97). Women who eat little or no red meat and vegetarians who eat no heme-iron foods and who do not regularly take iron supplements may enter pregnancy with less than adequate iron reserves.

Iron deficiency is hard to detect because your reserves will keep releasing iron to keep blood levels up. While tests that reveal blood levels can indicate the amount of iron in your reserves, it is hard to determine the true status of iron because iron production takes place in the bone marrow, and blood values don't easily reveal bone-marrow stores. Most women have low or virtually depleted iron reserves during the last trimester of pregnancy. Your doctor may measure red blood cells to determine your iron status. Iron deficiency is a progressive condition that can lead to anemia (see chapter 8).

Pica, a curious behavior in which women have a craving for a nonfood substance such as clay, dirt, laundry starch, cigarette ashes, milk of magnesia, cornstarch, coffee grounds, mothballs, erasers, or paint, is sometimes associated with low iron intake (202). There seems to be no common factor in these substances, and none of them contains iron, yet the cravings often stop when women are given iron supplements. Many women feel a sense of shame or guilt about eating such substances. Some believe that their baby will not be normal if these substances are not eaten. In some areas, tradition has it that eating clay ensures having beautiful children (19; 114), and the practice is passed from generation to generation.

The dangers of pica depend on the substance eaten—there can be bowel obstruction from clay or laundry starch, parasite infection from contaminated dirt, lead poisoning from painted plaster, and fetal blood disorders from chemicals in mothballs.

Mary had a friend who called her late one night in a panic. "I'm standing in my laundry room eating starch. I feel driven to eat it. What's going on? Am I crazy?" She was embarrassed to tell her doctor. Sure enough, she had stopped taking her iron supplements and hadn't told the doctor that, either. If she couldn't talk to her doctor, Mary counseled, it might be time to shop for a different doctor instead of a layette. When the iron supplements were restarted, her pica stopped, much to everyone's relief.

Some women crave ice cubes to alleviate the gum and tongue discomfort that can be caused by iron deficiency. This is one of the few instances in which specific nutrient deprivation is related to cravings during pregnancy.

Iron Supplements

"Iron is the only known nutrient for which requirements cannot be met reasonably by diet alone," the Subcommittee on Dietary Intake and Nutrient Supplements During Pregnancy writes, concurring with the 1989 Recommended Dietary Allowances. To meet the increased need for iron during the second and third trimesters of pregnancy, they advise pregnant women to take thirty milligrams of supplemental ferrous iron daily after the twelfth week of pregnancy in addition to the iron usually absorbed from food. High doses are not advised because they can impair absorption of zinc and other nutrients. Possible side effects from iron supplements are heartburn, nausea, constipation, and diarrhea (172).

Some women have fewer side effects if they take their iron

twice a day rather than in one larger dose. Others find it best if they take their iron supplement at bedtime. Research shows that iron in supplements is best absorbed if taken between meals. There are mixed reports on slow-release iron tablets; only those with proved effectiveness should be used. Iron absorption varies depending on what type of iron is used in a supplement. Some forms are more soluble than others.

GOOD IRON SOURCES

RDA during pregnancy: 30 milligrams per day
RDA during lactation: 15 milligrams per day

FOOD	PORTION	MILLIGRAMS IRON	CALORIES
Clams, canned, drained	¼ cup (1½ oz.)	11.8	64
Chili with beans, canned	1 cup	8.7	286
Chicken livers, cooked	3 oz.	7.3	135
Oysters, eastern	3 oz.	5.7	58
Beef liver, panfried	3 oz.	5.4	186
Baked beans w/pork, canned	1 cup	4.3	268
Liver sausage	2 oz.	3.4	177
Bean w/ham soup, chunky, canned	1 cup	3.2	231
Sirloin steak, lean broiled	3 oz.	2.9	178
Burrito, beef and bean	1, 6¼ oz.	2.7	392
Tuna, water packed	3 oz.	2.7	111
Ravioli, beef, canned	1 cup	2.3	223

FOOD	PORTION	MILLIGRAMS IRON	CALORIES
Macaroni or spaghetti, plain, enriched	1 cup	2.3	159
Hamburger, fast-food, w/bun	3 oz. patty	2.2	245
Lima beans, canned	½ cup	2.2	96
Waffle, frozen	1, 4″ square	1.7	95
English muffin	1 whole	1.6	135
Kidney beans, canned	½ cup	1.6	104
Turkey ham	2 oz.	1.6	73
Prune juice	½ cup	1.5	90
Spinach, frozen	½ cup	1.5	27
Fig bars	4	1.4	212
Tomato juice	1 cup	1.4	40
Peas	½ cup	1.3	63
Turkey, roast	3 oz.	1.2	135
Chicken, roast	3 oz.	1.0	163
Pita bread	1, 6½″	1.0	106
Prunes, dried	5 med.	1.0	100

Note: Dry and cooked cereals often have considerable added iron. Check nutrition labels.

IODINE AND FLUORIDE: ADDED PROTECTION

Iodine is a component of thyroxine, a substance produced by the thyroid gland located at the base of your throat. Your doctor checks the thyroid gland during a routine medical examination. *Thyroxine* regulates the rate at which the body uses energy. If iodine levels in the diet are low, thyroxine production falls. At the same time, the thyroid gland may enlarge, creating a condition called *goiter*. Until iodized salt was introduced in 1924, iodine-deficiency goiter was common in certain areas of the United States; now it is very rare in this country. Foods grown in soil that is near salt-water oceans contain iodine; so do animals that graze on grass near oceans. Ocean fish are also a good source of iodine. Because food processing equipment is cleaned with solutions that contain iodine, the mineral is transferred to many processed foods.

The RDA for iodine for adult women is 150 micrograms. During pregnancy, an additional 25 micrograms is recommended to meet fetal needs, so the RDA for pregnancy is 175 micrograms per day. The average intake by women twenty-five to thirty years old in this country is 170 micrograms per day (136). Eating iodized salt to taste on foods should take care of the increased need for iodine during pregnancy.

Be cautious about taking iodine-containing asthma medications when you are pregnant. Check with your doctor about this and all prescribed medications. The very large doses of iodine that some of these medications contain have been reported to induce an iodine imbalance and thyroid-gland problems in the newborn (85).

Fluoride is an important mineral with a starring role in public controversy. While fluoridation efforts are directed primarily to children under age sixteen, adults may benefit from a fluoridated water supply or a one-milligram-per-day supplement to prevent tooth decay (58).

Fluoride bonds calcium and phosphorus in bones and teeth. It helps to make teeth strong and resistant to decay. Tooth decay in children has been reduced by about 40 percent in communities that have added fluoride to water at the level of one part per million (1 ppm) (25). One part per million is a very tiny amount, equivalent to a few drops in a swimming pool.

Fluoride is naturally present in some water, usually well water, and in amounts in excess of 1 ppm in some places. Excessive fluoride can cause discolored spots on teeth, which, while not physically harmful, aren't cosmetically attractive.

If you live in an area that does not have fluoridated water, ask your dentist about fluoride treatments for you and your family. Bottled water with added fluoride is also available.

Fetal formation of the tooth system begins at about the tenth week of pregnancy. Four permanent molars and eight incisors begin developing between the sixth and ninth months (202). Because there is little calcium in these preeruptive teeth, the effect of fluoride may be negligible. One study done in 1982 suggests that taking fluoride during pregnancy does help prevent tooth decay in childhood (72). But since these findings have not been validated, the American Dental Association does not, at this time, endorse prenatal fluoride supplements (172).

ZINC

Zinc is important to digestion, metabolism, breathing, wound healing, and maintenance of skin and hair. It is part of more than two hundred enzymes and many hormones. During pregnancy, zinc plays an important role in the formation of the developing organs, skeleton, and internal systems like nerves and circulation. Since zinc is essential to reproduction, dietary zinc becomes especially important during pregnancy (202).

People get about 70 percent of their zinc from animal foods. Like iron, zinc is better absorbed from animal than from vegetable sources (36). Since meat is a major source of the mineral, vegetarians may have a hard time getting adequate zinc. Tobacco and alcohol interfere with zinc absorption (172). Taking zinc supplements will not change the recommendation to give up these substances during pregnancy.

A daily zinc supplement of fifty milligrams can impair copper and iron metabolism (104). Supplements containing more than twice the recommended daily amount of iron per day can lower zinc absorption (43).

Zinc toxicity is rare, though megadoses are becoming more common as zinc gains popularity as a self-help remedy for a variety of problems. Premature and stillborn births have been reported, although not confirmed, by one research study of women who took large doses of supplementary zinc during the last few months of pregnancy (9). Mothers who took megadoses of zinc are much more likely to give birth to babies with birth defects (99).

The best way to get enough zinc, but not too much, is to be aware of good sources of zinc and include them in your diet. A good varied diet that does not rely too much on processed foods will provide zinc.

Is it true what they say about oysters? Oysters *are* the very best source of zinc. The connection between zinc and virility accounts for the reputation they enjoy as an aphrodisiac. Although severe zinc deficiencies may result in retarded sexual growth, and although it has been shown that zinc can be used to treat impotency in men who lose zinc through kidney dialysis, zinc cannot cure general impotence. Since impotency is not a problem associated with pregnancy, this may not be of concern to you, but it does make eating oysters more enjoyable and will certainly make good table conversation!

Although oysters are a zinc bonanza, be careful what you eat. Do not eat raw oysters. Food poisoning can be particularly dangerous during pregnancy. Eat your oysters in stew, simmered, or even fried—on a diet that allows moderate amounts of fat, there is room for an occasional fried food. A New Orleans oyster sandwich (fried oysters on French bread with lettuce, tomatoes, and a bit of tartar and Tabasco sauce) can be a real treat!

GOOD ZINC SOURCES

RDA in pregnancy: 15 milligrams per day
RDA in lactation; first 6 months, 19 milligrams per day; second 6 months, 16 milligrams per day

FOOD	PORTION	MILLIGRAMS ZINC
Oysters, Eastern	3 oz.	84.0
Oysters, Pacific	3 oz.	14.0
Oyster stew, canned, prepared w/milk	1 cup	10.3
Calves liver, panfried	3 oz.	6.7
Chili with beans, canned	1 cup	5.1
Beef liver, panfried	3 oz.	4.6

FOOD	PORTION	MILLIGRAMS ZINC
Beef, sirloin, lean, cooked	3 oz.	4.4
Lamb, leg, lean, roasted	3 oz.	4.2
Turkey, dark meat, roasted	3 oz.	3.8
Baked beans, vegetarian, canned	1 cup	3.6
Cheeseburger, fast-food, w/bun	3 oz. patty	2.5
Bean burrito	1, 6 oz.	2.4
Chicken, dark meat, cooked	3 oz.	2.4
Spaghetti sauce w/meat, homemade	1 cup	2.1
Cheese pizza, regular crust	1 slice, 5 oz.	2.0
Yogurt, plain, lowfat	1 cup	2.0
Sunflower seeds, dried	$\frac{1}{4}$ cup	1.8
Turkey breast, roasted	3 oz.	1.7
Rye wafers, whole grain	2	1.6
Pork chop, panfried	1, 3 oz.	1.4
Black-eyed peas	$\frac{1}{2}$ cup	1.3
Garbanzo beans, canned	$\frac{1}{2}$ cup	1.3
Shrimp, boiled	3 oz.	1.3
Split pea soup w/ham, canned	1 cup	1.3
Macaroni and cheese	1 cup	1.2
Oatmeal	1 cup	1.2
Perch, baked	3 oz.	1.2
Chicken, light meat	3 oz.	1.1
Milk, 1%, 2%, or buttermilk	1 cup	1.0

COPPER: A HIDDEN TREASURE?

A pregnant woman has twice the level of copper in her blood as a nonpregnant woman does (76). The scientific explanation is not yet clear. And yet, to date, most research on copper has been done with men (172). Copper is among the nutrients named by the Subcommittee on Dietary Intake and Nutrient Supplements requiring further study in relation to pregnancy (172).

What is known is that copper plays key roles in making red blood cells, the sheath around nerves, and connective tissues, and it assists in the production of energy and the respiration process. On the basis of weight, the brain is the most concentrated site of copper. A fetus builds up stores of copper in its liver late in pregnancy to sustain it during the first two to three months after birth (145).

Copper deficiency during human pregnancy is virtually unknown because copper is widely available in foods and water. This is indeed fortunate since copper-deficient lab animals are more likley to give birth to malformed offspring (93). Copper levels in the blood are lower in women who deliver prematurely (101). Zinc can interfere with copper absorption, but if copper is added to zinc supplements, it reduces the interference (174).

The best sources of copper are whole grains, shellfish (especially crabmeat), liver and kidney, raisins, nuts, peas and beans, and fresh fruits and vegetables.

One note of caution: Acid foods, especially slowly cooked ones like spaghetti sauce, can contain dangerously high levels of copper if prepared in copper cookware. Cooking in copper pots can destroy vitamins C, E, and folacin. If you use copper pans, be sure they are well-lined. There is no problem with copper-bottomed stainless steel pots.

MORE TRACE MINERALS

Other trace minerals (molybdenum, cobalt, manganese, and selenium) are essential to human life, but little is known about their functions specific to pregnancy. Following the eating game plan in chapter 3 will help you meet your needs for vitamins and minerals—even those we know very little about. For now, the best advice we can give is to eat a variety of foods.

7

Playing It Safe

QUICK QUIZ

The answers are within this chapter and on page 294.

True or False

___ 1. Pregnant women are more susceptible to food poisoning than nonpregnant women.
___ 2. You can get food poisoning from eating rare meat.
___ 3. Pregnant women can eat any amount of fish, as long as the fish is from local waters.
___ 4. A cup of instant tea has more caffeine than a cup of freshly brewed tea.
___ 5. Alcohol is most dangerous during the third trimester of pregnancy.
___ 6. *Heavy drinking* is generally defined as two or more drinks a day.
___ 7. Low-tar and -nicotine cigarettes reduce risks to an unborn child.
___ 8. Some cough syrups and cold remedies contain substantial amounts of alcohol.
___ 9. Pregnant women should not take aspirin.
___ 10. Cigarette smoking is the single greatest cause of poor fetal growth in developed countries.

Women have carried babies through wars and storms and periods of severe social and economic deprivation over which they had no control. This chapter is about the safety of a prenatal environment that you *can* control.

FOOD THAT'S SAFE TO EAT

Food Poisoning

Tens of millions of Americans experience food poisoning every year (53). During pregnancy, you are even more vulnerable to food-borne microorganisms and more likely to have severe reactions (71). The prolonged diarrhea or vomiting that accompanies food poisoning can lead to dehydration, fluid imbalance, and loss of nutrients. In addition, medications used to treat some types of food-borne illnesses are not suitable for use during pregnancy.

You cannot see, smell, or taste food-borne bacteria, and many foods virtually always contain bacteria. It's when there are dangerous kinds or huge amounts of bacteria that we become sick. Proper heating will destroy most bacteria, but if the bacteria have already multiplied and produced poisons, some of these toxins are not destroyed even by heat (71). Thus, keeping bacteria from multiplying reduces the risk of food-borne illness.

Food poisoning does not result only from eating at a picnic, in a restaurant with a dirty kitchen, or from a quaint street vendor in an exotic part of the world.

Many home kitchens would not pass a food safety and sanitation test. Now is a good time to learn the basics on safe food handling.

- Wash your hands before you begin preparing food.

- Make sure foods are clean. Thoroughly wash or peel fruits and vegetables before you eat them.
- Take care when handling uncooked chicken and other meats. Use soap and hot water to wash and rinse every surface that comes into contact with the meat (sink, counter, cutting board, knife). If you cut up chicken and then prepare a salad with the same knife, you may contaminate the salad with *Campylobacter jejuni* or *Salmonella* bacteria from the raw chicken. Unfortunately, most chickens carry *Salmonella*. These microorganisms occur naturally in our environment. Always cook chicken thoroughly before eating it.
- Keep hot foods hot (at least 140° F) and cold foods cold (at most 40° F). If you buy hot carryout foods, bring them directly home and reheat or refrigerate them immediately. Don't order ready-to-eat foods and let them stand on the counter for several hours before dinner. Always refrigerate leftovers immediately after a meal—nasty food microbes love a warm, moist environment. If you prepare food in large quantities, don't leave it out to cool; divide it into several shallow pans for quick cooling in the refrigerator or freezer. Meat and other perishables should be transported quickly to your refrigerator or freezer. If you're running errands on the way home from the supermarket, put perishables in an insulated carrier in your car. Party and picnic perishables should be at room temperature no more than two hours. On a buffet, put out small quantities, replenish often from refrigerated or hot reserves, and discard leftover food that has been sitting out. This is not wasteful—it's good food-safety sense!

- Everybody, whether pregnant or not, should avoid raw milk (unpasteurized), foods prepared with raw or undercooked eggs (soft-cooked eggs, Caesar salad, homemade ice cream and mayonnaise, eggnog, desserts made with whipped egg whites), uncooked meat (very rare meat, steak tartare), and raw fish (sushi, raw oysters or clams, lightly steamed mussels or snails).
- Eggs, seafood, and meat should always be well cooked before eating. There are increasing reports of viral and parasitic infections traced to eating raw seafood (39). Put raw meat, fish, and poultry in plastic bags so drippings won't contaminate other foods. Use pasteurized eggnog, baked meringues, and bottled Caesar salad dressing rather than freshly made versions containing raw eggs.
- Many of us wouldn't admit it, but we often snitch ice cream, cottage cheese, peanut butter, or fruit juice right out of the container. Bacteria from your mouth contaminates food. For the same reason, don't dip vegetables or chips again after you've taken a bite, and don't share dips with other people.

Food Additives—An Added Risk?

Food additives and fetuses just don't sound as though they belong in the same womb. Most of us have learned to accept a little sodium propionate in our bread and a judicious bit of propylene glycol monostearate in our salad dressing, but what happens to an unborn child when it gets a dose of an antimicrobial additive or emulsifier?

Government regulatory agencies require that new food

additives be tested to simulate situations that could produce ill effects. If the additive is deemed safe, regulations are established for the types of foods in which it can be used, the maximum quantities that can be used, and the way it must be described on the label. Food additives are more tightly regulated now than at any other time in history.

Rather than being harmful, some additives protect food quality and safety. Others add color or flavor. Nevertheless, you may have concerns about additives that have made headlines from time to time: nitrites, artificial colors and flavors, monosodium glutamate (MSG), artificial sweeteners, and fats. Most people's concern about them has to do with cancer. What do we know about their safety during pregnancy?

NITRITES

Nitrites are added to cured meats to maintain their color and prevent them from developing the potentially dangerous toxin botulin. Nitrites can be converted to nitrosamines (see below) when bacon is fried at very high temperatures. Other cured fish, meats, and several vegetables also contain some nitrites. The presence of vitamin C inhibits nitrites from forming nitrosamines, so vitamin C is sometimes added to cured foods.

NITROSAMINES

Nitrosamines are of legitimate concern as possible carcinogens, but whether they pose a risk to an unborn child has not been determined. Our advice: Limit cured meats, fish, and bacon, and don't cook with bacon drippings, which are even higher in nitrosamines. Bacon, hot dogs, and cured cold cuts aren't on the Best Choices food lists for pregnancy anyway.

Don't worry about occasional use or small amounts of these foods. Just don't eat them daily.

SULFITES

Sulfites present problems to some people, particularly those with asthma. Between 5 and 10 percent of persons with asthma may be sensitive to sulfites, and their reactions can be severe. Sulfiting agents are used to maintain a fresh appearance and stop light-colored fruits and vegetables from darkening. Their use on salad bar ingredients was banned in 1986. The Food and Drug Administration (FDA) requires labeling on foods that contain sulfites. Processed potatoes, many dried fruits (like light raisins and dried pears), and some beer and wine contain sulfites.

ARTIFICIAL COLORS AND FLAVORS

Artificial colors and flavors have been extensively studied. In 1960, there were two hundred colors used in foods; now there are only thirty-three approved by the FDA (155). The FDA says that no artificial color or flavor can be used if it covers up spoilage.

About 10 percent of all food eaten in the United States contains certified food colors (36). The soft drink industry is the largest user of certified colors, but cereals, candies, snack foods, gelatins, desserts, ice creams, and many baked goods contain certified colors too (36).

A few people (one or two in ten thousand) are allergic to *FD&C Yellow No. 5* (tartrazine). If you are one of these people, you probably know of your sensitivity before pregnancy. The symptoms of tartrazine allergy are itching, hives, nasal congestion, and headaches (87). This additive is always labeled when it is used in a food. Common food sources of tartrazine include orange drinks, gelatin, processed cheese dinners, cake mixes, and snacks. Artificial colors or flavors have not been correlated with any birth defects or complications specific to pregnancy.

Monosodium glutamate (MSG) is a chemical used as a flavor enhancer. MSG is frequently used in preparing Chinese foods, but you can generally request that restaurants prepare food without MSG. Some individuals are especially sensitive to MSG. If you have developed symptoms such as headache, nausea, vomiting, or dizziness after eating the additive, it would be best to avoid all foods with MSG whether or not you are pregnant. MSG, which is also an ingredient of hydrolized plant protein, will have mandatory labeling within the next year.

SUGAR SUBSTITUTES

Saccharin, cyclamates, and aspartame are sugar substitutes. Cyclamates are not currently sold in the United States, but are widely used in Canada. Saccharin and aspartame are commonly used in low-calorie and dietetic products in the United States. Saccharin was the first artificial sweetener and has been used for almost one hundred years. Aspartame, a chemical compound 180 times sweeter than sugar, was approved by the FDA in 1981.

The safety of all sugar substitutes has been questioned repeatedly in the scientific literature. In amounts normally used, all of the sweeteners are probably safe. Used in huge quantities, however, they have harmed a few laboratory rats.

When aspartame was introduced there were many consumer concerns about its safety. Intense research by manufacturers determined that aspartame creates no serious widespread safety problem, although some individuals may have a sensitivity to it. Long-term and case-controlled studies are now under way.

Individuals who have a genetic metabolic disorder known as phenylketonuria (PKU) build up large amounts of phenylalanine—one of the amino acids found in aspartame—in their blood. This condition doesn't happen unless you have PKU, and if you do, you know it and have been on a special diet all your life. Individuals who have PKU should avoid aspartame. A buildup of phenylalanine during pregnancy can damage the fetal brain (202). Individuals who do not have PKU would have to have the equivalent of sixty twelve-ounce cans of an aspartame-containing soft drink at one time to create a harmful concentration in the blood. A pregnant woman would have to drink one can of diet soda every eight minutes, twenty-four hours a day, to produce a dangerously high blood level of phenylalanine. Since this is physically impossible, there is no reason to suggest that pregnant women strictly avoid aspartame (171).

If you are diabetic, eating foods containing sugar substitutes instead of sugar is wise. But most pregnant women should be conservative in their use of foods high in nonnutritive sweeteners and other chemical ingredients. Many of these new ingredients have not been around long enough for us to know whether there are long-term effects on humans.

We asked Julie Scheier, a registered dietitian at Prentice Women's Hospital in Chicago, how she responds to questions about diet soda (159). She counsels pregnant women to restrict diet soft drinks to two per day if they drink diet soda at all. Ask your doctor or dietitian about an appropriate amount if you regularly drink diet soda. There's no need to consume large amounts of nonnutritive sweeteners during pregnancy. After all, dieting is not advisable and caffeine consumption should be limited. Nutrient-rich milk and fruit juices are the beverages of choice.

Other fabricated products will become part of our food supply in the years to come. Any new product will have passed rigid safety tests, but only the test of time can show absolute safety. Since healthful alternatives are available, we advise taking a cautious approach during pregnancy.

To avoid excessive additives

- Limit processed and fabricated foods and foods made from packaged mixes
- Use fresh meat and poultry instead of processed cold cuts and smoked meat
- Choose fresh fruit and dairy products instead of packaged snacks
- Drink water and lowfat milk instead of regular or diet soft drinks
- Read ingredient listings on food labels

Information on food safety is available from the National Center for Nutrition and Dietetics, the public education initiative of the American Dietetic Association and its Foundation. Write to: NDND, 216 Jackson Boulevard, Suite 800, Chicago, IL 60606. Ask for booklets on food storage, food-borne illness, or food additives. A registered dietitian is available to answer nutrition questions. This is a free service—just call 1-800-366-1655. NCND can also give you the name of a registered dietitian who does individual counseling in you community.

Pesticides and Food Contaminants

Thanks to stricter regulations and the vigilance of consumer groups, our food supply is growing increasingly safe. Use of many pesticides (DDT, dieldrin, heptachlor, chlordane) has been suspended by the Environmental Protection Agency; others, such as alar and EDB, are carefully regulated and monitored (36). Surveys conducted by the FDA show that levels of pesticides in foods are generally very low. These surveys show that most residues are in fats and oils of meat, fish, and poultry. Legumes and vegetables have the fewest residues. Fruits were found to have the greatest variety of chemical residues. You are not likely to encounter dangerously high levels of herbicides in commercially grown foods, and you can avoid dioxin and toxic malathion in home gardening.

Because environmental residues (PCBs, PBBs, etc.) can get into water supplies, we recommend that pregnant women limit eating freshwater fish caught by sport fishermen. Check with your local department of health or state department of fisheries about the safety of local lakes and streams. Bait shops, where fishing licenses are sold, may be able to provide you with information. Ask for your state's fishing regulations.

Heavy metals, including mercury, lead, cadmium, and possibly nickel and selenium, can be toxic in sufficient amounts, but there is not much actual risk to you. There are reports of localized environmental exposure in specific areas when local water supplies are contaminated. Local water supplies can also be chemically contaminated when highly toxic herbicides (chlorinated dioxin, Agent Orange) are sprayed in forested areas. Continual vigilance is needed by individuals, environmental groups, and government agencies to protect us from dangerous substances.

But some perspective is needed, too. In the late 1980s, the public became aware of a potential problem with alar, a chemical used in apple orchards. Alar is a systemic insecticide sprayed on trees. The media boosted public concern to hysteria that was unwarranted based on scientific evidence. Use of alar in the United States is now restricted. In retrospect, however, despite great public alarm, there was no real risk in the amount of alar used and not even one report of damage to a human being.

If you are concerned about pesticides, trim visible fat, eat less fatty fish, and peel fruits and vegetables. If fruits and vegetables cannot be peeled, carefully wash them with dish soap, rinsing well, to remove dirt and chemical residues. To preserve nutrients and help stored produce last longer, wash it before you eat it rather than before refrigerating it.

CAFFEINE

Coffee and tea are among the most popular beverages in the world. In the United States, 1.74 cups of coffee were consumed per person per day in 1986 (36). Tea is regularly consumed by 31 percent of the population. Coffee and tea are the greatest contributors to caffeine intake, although soft drinks and chocolate also provide caffeine. How much each source supplies depends on an individual's habits.

CAFFEINE COUNTER

FOOD	PORTION	MILLIGRAMS CAFFEINE
Chocolate		
bar (Cadbury/Hershey)	1 oz.	15–20
baking chocolate (Bakers)	1 oz.	25
chocolate milk	8 oz.	4–8
Cocoa, hot chocolate	1 cup	6–42
cocoa, dry	1 tbsp.	15
Coffee, brewed	1 cup (8 oz.)	128
instant	1 rnd. tsp.	60
decaffeinated	1 cup	3
powdered, flavored	6 oz.	41–50
Desserts		
pudding pops	1 bar	1–3
chocolate pudding	½ cup	4–12
Drugs		
Aspirin*	1 tab.	30–32/pill
Cope, Midol	1 tab.	30–32/pill
Exedrin, Anacin, Pre-Mens	1 tab.	60–66/pill
No Doz, Vivarin	1 tab.	100–200/pill
cold preparations*	1 tab.	30–100/pill
Soft drinks, cola, diet cola		
Coke, Pepsi, RC	12 oz.	32–65
Tab	12 oz.	46
Dr. Pepper	12 oz.	37
Mountain Dew, Mr. Pibb	12 oz.	40–54
7-Up, Sprite	12 oz.	0
Tea (brewed 3 minutes)		
green	6 oz.	40
black	8 oz.	60
instant	1 tsp.	30

*Some, not all, of these preparations contain caffeine. Check the labels.

Caffeine passes quickly into the human bloodstream, ready to stimulate your tired brain and muscles—and your baby. Caffeine crosses the placenta, and because fetal organs cannot process it well, the stimulant becomes concentrated in the fetal bloodstream (6). Drinking more than two cups of coffee can also change maternal hormone levels and blood flow to the placenta (102).

Scientists offer conflicting advice about the safety or danger of caffeine. Large quantities of caffeine (equivalent to twenty to one hundred cups of coffee a day) have produced birth defects and low birth weight in rats, mice, rabbits, and chickens. But the prevailing view supported by a recent study of 12,000 women is that there is no convincing evidence that caffeine is associated with birth defects or reduced birth weight in humans (172). Because negative effects can be produced in several animal species, and because the seriousness of defects can be correlated with the amounts of caffeine given, some researchers feel there is ample reason to send up the yellow warning flag for pregnant women. Others point out that animals and human beings metabolize caffeine differently (197), that studies indicate risk only from very large quantities of caffeine, and that the effects of smaller quantities of caffeine have not been determined (202).

In 1980, the surgeon general of the United States and the FDA advised pregnant women to use caffeine products sparingly (110). Since that warning, it has been reported that women who consume more than 150 milligrams of caffeine daily (one and a half cups of coffee) may increase their risk of miscarriage (170). In contrast, many studies have reported that moderate consumption of caffeine during pregnancy has no adverse effects on the fetus (172).

Caffeine is thought to promote increased excretion of calcium and decreased zinc and iron absorption (117). Tea and coffee contain acids that can irritate the digestive tract. Caffeine stimulates secretion of acid in the stomach, promoting indigestion and heartburn. Kidneys produce more urine when high levels of caffeine are present, causing loss of fluids, vitamins, and minerals (118).

And we all know about caffeine and sleep. As pregnancy progresses, your bumping, thrashing, bulging baby will sometimes make it hard to get a good night's sleep. Neither you nor baby needs more stimulation. A nice glass of milk, not coffee, will help put both you and baby to sleep.

Tea

If you are feeling smug because you drink tea, you may be in for a surprise. While most teas contain less caffeine than coffee, many do contain significant amounts. The tea connoisseur who likes loose, imported tea in a full-strength brew is the one most likely to get the heavy dose of caffeine. The bag-in-bag-out drinker gets considerably less caffeine in her cup.

Herbal teas, the beverage of choice for many who avoid caffeine, may not be the sweet, innocent health drinks they purport to be. Julie Scheier, R.D., points out that while popular brands of no-caffeine teas contain only ingredients considered to be safe, herbal teas from health food stores or mail-order sources can be harmful (159). Some "natural" herbs and tea materials such as sassafras and mistletoe have major pharmacologic effects that can be dangerous during pregnancy. Some contain substances that can cause vomiting, diarrhea, heart palpitations, lowered blood pressure, and allergic reactions.

While some herbal teas such as bittersweet, horsechestnut, and spotted hemlock contain known toxins, they are not likely to be banned by the Food and Drug Administration because these substances are naturally occurring, not added during processing. It is unwise, and may be unsafe, to use herbal teas packaged without adequate ingredient information on the label. Advice about the benefits of ingredients in herbal teas often does not stand up to scientific or medical scrutiny. While there is no research specifically related to their effects on the fetus, herbal teas (especially unregulated blends) should be considered druglike, and drugs are always viewed as questionable during pregnancy. Julie Scheier advises her patients to limit even trusted herbal tea to two cups a day.

Decaffeination

Many people have decided to give up or cut back on caffeine, and a wide assortment of decaffeinated coffee, tea, and soft drinks is now available. Decaffeinating reduces caffeine in coffee and tea to virtually nothing, but some of the acids that cause indigestion and heartburn remain. Taking the caffeine out of coffee does not remove other substances that may be harmful during pregnancy.

Because there have been few studies on decaffeinated products, there may be effects on mother and baby that we do not yet understand. Caffeine can be removed from coffee and tea either with methylene chloride or with a nonchemical water process. Though very little of the methylene chloride remains after processing some people prefer water-processed brands. Brands change rapidly, so read the label to find out which are water processed.

The caffeine removed in decaffeinating coffee beans does not necessarily go to waste. Some may be recycled into soft drinks. At one time, the FDA Standards of Identity required that when beverages called themselves cola or pepper drinks, they had to contain caffeine. Drinking a caffeine-charged cola to get going in the morning is becoming increasingly popular, and manufacturers are responding by introducing new caffeine-fortified colas.

Chocolate

Though we cannot blame caffeine for the "addiction" some people seem to have for chocolate, there are significant amounts in chocolate products. Chocolate's active ingredient is theobromine, a substance that has physiologic effects and a chemical structure similar to caffeine, but its action on the nervous system is slightly different. A typical cup of cocoa contains less than twenty milligrams of caffeine but more than two hundred milligrams of theobromine. Chocolate also creates certain physiologic effects, causing release of brain chemicals associated with pleasure or relaxation.

Over-the-Counter Drugs

Over-the-counter drugs can be another major source of caffeine. Caffeine is used in cold remedies because it dilates blood vessels. It's a stimulant that wards off sleep and counteracts depression. In diet pills, caffeine elevates blood sugar. Since the effects of caffeine are related to body weight, a fetus may be endangered. Any drug not specifically prescribed by your doctor should be avoided, regardless of its caffeine content.

CUTTING BACK

The chart on page 201 will help you determine how much caffeine you consume. If the amount is high enough to warrant altering your habits, try these methods of limiting caffeine.

- Count the cups or mugs of coffee or tea you drink to avoid casual overconsumption.
- Switch to a small cup instead of a large mug.
- Choose beverages that contain no caffeine.
- Reduce caffeine by drinking decaffeinated coffee, tea, and soft drinks.
- Avoid taking medications with caffeine; take no medications without your doctor's advice.

There's not enough data to point to a strict, specific limit on caffeine for pregnant women. There is enough evidence, though, to advise limiting coffee during pregnancy (126). Switch to lowfat milk, fruit juices, and mineral water as much as possible. If you continue to consume caffeine, it makes sense to limit your intake (172).

Be aware of how you define a "cup" of coffee. The mug on your desk may contain a good bit more than the six-ounce portion in a traditional cup of coffee: Measure it and you may find that *your* cup is, in fact, ten ounces of coffee! Similarly, the number of these cups you drink in a day (or night) may not be clear-cut. Many of us would be hard-pressed to count, because we add a little to the cup to warm it up every time we pass the pot. Those of us who have access to a continual supply are the most likely to get hooked on this habit.

If you abruptly cut back on caffeine, you may experience unpleasant symptoms of withdrawal such as headache, nervousness, or irritability. One way to avoid these reactions is to mix decaffeinated coffee or tea with your regular brand, gradually increasing the proportion of the decaffeinated product until you have adjusted to the new taste and level of stimulation. It may make it a little harder to "get going" in the morning, but you and baby will sleep better at night!

ALCOHOL AND THE UNBORN CHILD

In ancient Sparta, young married couples were forbidden alcohol because they found it produced less than healthy babies. The Bible warns pregnant women not to drink alcohol (15). Historically pregnancy has carried with it restrictions about alcohol consumption. Now, on behalf of your baby, we present the following information.

Ethyl alcohol (the alcohol found in beer, wines, and distilled spirits) affects your body in ways no other substance does. First, ethyl alcohol is absorbed more quickly than any of the nutrients. It is rapidly transported to the liver, where it is processed and changed into energy at the rate of seven calories per gram (compare that to four calories per gram in carbohydrates and protein and nine calories per gram in fats). These calories are limited in their usefulness, however.

The liver can handle only limited amounts of ethyl alcohol at a time. It can completely process only about a third of an ounce of alcohol an hour; that's an hour and a half to metabolize the alcohol in one drink or a twelve-ounce can of beer! If you eat as you drink, and sip your drink over a long period of time, you may be able to slow down the rate of absorption and keep alcohol at a level that can be processed by the liver. If an overload occurs, the excess alcohol circulates in the bloodstream until the liver can handle it. Some is excreted; some evaporates as it passes through the lung (and can be smelled on a person's breath). While in the bloodstream, it affects every organ it passes.

Alcohol goes through the placenta and into the circulatory system of the fetus (133). It affects every organ there, too. The fetal brain is growing at a rate of one hundred thousand new brain cells a minute, so deprivation of oxygen to the brain or the umbilical cord for even a few moments can have a negative impact. A sudden rise in alcohol in the bloodstream can halt delivery of oxygen through the umbilical cord (192).

In 1981, the Surgeon General's Advisory included a warning that still stands: "Women who are pregnant or even considering pregnancy should avoid alcohol completely and should be aware of the alcoholic content of food and drugs" (175). That "even considering pregnancy" is important because many women do not know they are pregnant in the first few weeks, a period of rapid cell division and a time of very high vulnerability for the fetus. The American Medical Association agrees, advising women to stop drinking as soon as they *plan* to become pregnant.

The surgeon general's conservative approach grows out of studies demonstrating that, while women who have five or more drinks a day are most at risk, even moderate drinking is associated with retarded fetal growth and an increased rate of spontaneous abortions (144). A study in 1984 showed significant risk of delivering a growth-retarded infant for women who had only one to two drinks a day (122).

EQUIVALENT AMOUNTS OF ALCOHOL *(ABOUT 0.5 OUNCE PURE ALCOHOL)*

One drink is

1 jigger, $1\frac{1}{2}$ oz.	Spirits: whiskey, rum, gin, vodka, scotch, etc.
1 glass, 5 oz.	Wine: dry table wine, red or white
1 glass, 10 oz.	Beer
1 glass, 12 oz.	Beer: light types

Heavy drinking during pregnancy, defined as two or more drinks a day, is now the leading cause of mental and physical retardation, surpassing Downs syndrome (186). About one in 750 children born in the United States is a victim of this preventable damage (192). When five or more ounces of alcohol are consumed daily, there is a great possibility of fetal alcohol syndrome. The term *fetal alcohol syndrome* (FAS) was first used in 1973 to describe a recognizable pattern of physical and mental birth defects in many babies born to women who are very heavy drinkers or chronic alcoholics.

Babies with FAS are abnormally small at birth, especially in head size, and do not have the same amount of brain tissue as normal children do. Since alcohol prevents cell division and growth, the brain simply does not develop to fill out the head. The eyes are too close together and are covered by a fold of skin at the inner corners; there is virtually no bridge to the nose and the space above the lip is flat. The affected children are severely mentally retarded and usually have emotional problems; about half have heart defects, and many have abnormal internal organs.

Many of these babies are irritable and jittery in the first few days after birth as they begin their lives in alcohol withdrawal. As they grow, they exhibit behavioral problems, short attention spans, and poor coordination (94).

Not every mother who drinks heavily gives birth to a baby with FAS, and not every FAS baby has all the defects. The effects of alcohol consumption may be more subtle and not result in full FAS, but cause mild to moderate mental and physical retardation, inability to concentrate, hyperactivity, and behavioral or sleep problems that are not apparent until the child grows older. This is called *fetal alcohol effects* (FAE) or *modified FAS*.

Alcohol can also indirectly affect fetal development by interfering with maternal nutrition. Women who drink large quantities of alcohol get a substantial portion of calories from alcohol and may have little appetite for other more nutritious foods. Vitamins, especially thiamin and niacin, are used to process alcohol in the liver and so their stores are depleted. In addition, drinking often causes increased excretion and urination, flushing vitamins, minerals, and fluids out of the mother's body.

Heavy drinkers tend to be deficient in two very important nutrients for pregnancy—iron and folacin. Alcohol may also interfere with placental transport of amino acids, the protein building blocks of fetal tissue. Multivitamin-mineral supplementation is recommended for women who are heavy drinkers, but supplements will not counteract the effects of alcohol.

Cutting Down

We all know women who have continued to drink moderately during pregnancy and who have had perfectly normal, healthy children. If you drank before you discovered you were pregnant or before you read this book, worrying won't help. Take action now to give your baby the best possible environment in which to grow from today on.

If you're a light or moderate drinker, try to avoid alcohol altogether, whether it's from a glass of wine or from cough syrup. Your body doesn't know whether the alcohol you drink comes from a martini, a beer, a cold remedy, or a brandy-flamed dessert. You may be surprised to learn that alcohol does not completely evaporate when it is cooked or flamed: A study done at Washington State University showed that alcoholic beverages retain as much as 85 percent of their alcohol after cooking (24). A sauce made with burgundy retained 5 percent of its alcohol after two and a half hours of cooking; another wine sauce, simmered for ten minutes, retained 40 percent of its alcohol. Baked scalloped oysters still had 45 percent of the alcohol from added sherry, and flaming cherries jubilee burned away only 25 percent of the alcohol. These data are enough to warrant other choices by pregnant women.

Some mouthwashes, cough syrups, and cold remedies contain substantial amounts of alcohol. To avoid alcohol-containing preparations, read the label or ask the pharmacist.

If you're a heavy drinker, just because no one sees you drunk, you never miss work, and don't drink before noon does not mean that you are not a problem drinker. Now, every drink you take makes a difference to your baby. If you find that you cannot control your drinking, we hope that the prospect of having a less-than-able child will give you the courage to seek help. Alcoholism is a disease that, like other diseases, needs treatment—and special care during pregnancy.

THE SMOKE-FILLED WOMB

Cigarette smoking is the single most modifiable determinant of poor fetal growth and subsequent reduced birth weight in the developed world (103). Some 15 to 30 percent of women in the United States smoke cigarettes at the time of their first prenatal visit (186). Women who smoke give birth to babies weighing an average of about a half pound less than nonsmoking women.

Maternal smoking during pregnancy

- Increases metabolic rate, making fewer calories available for fetal growth (139)
- Increases iron and vitamin C requirements (172)
- Interferes with absorption and utilization of folate, zinc, vitamins B_{12} and C, and amino acids (172)
- Reduces maternal-placental blood flow, thus restricting nutrients and oxygen to the fetus (172)
- Puts cyanide, a constituent of tobacco smoke, into the bloodstream of the fetus; nutrients are used to detoxify the cyanide
- Increases the likelihood of miscarriage (57)
- Results in 50 percent more premature deliveries than among nonsmoking mothers and more than twice as many low-birth-weight babies (10)

- Doubles a woman's risk of having a stillborn baby (183)
- May have long-term effects on the child's mental and physical well-being (128)

Understanding the true long-term effects of maternal smoking is complicated by the fact that the baby, once born, usually lives in an environment contaminated by smoke.

How Much You Smoke Makes a Difference

The birth weight of babies is influenced by the number of cigarettes smoked, and even light smoking (five or six cigarettes a day) results in babies that weigh (on average) less than those of nonsmoking mothers (10).

The nicotine in cigarettes speeds up your heartbeat by ten to twenty beats a minute, and even one cigarette can produce a sudden speeding-up, then slowing-down of the fetal heartbeat (10). Nicotine also causes arteries to constrict and makes arteries in the wall of the uterus contract, reducing the flow of blood to the placenta. If this happens, some of the cells in the uterus may die and the attachment between the placenta and the uterus can weaken. This condition is thought to be the reason for the increased rate of spontaneous abortions and preterm deliveries among women who smoke.

The March of Dimes says that mothers who stop smoking or significantly reduce their smoking by the fifth month of pregnancy can spare their babies possible damage (115). Stopping smoking is a great gift to your baby, to yourself, and to the health of other family members.

Low-Tar and -Nicotine Cigarettes

Low-tar and -nicotine cigarettes may be less harmful than regular cigarettes, but they're still not good enough for pregnancy (183). They produce carbon monoxide, which slows down the flow of oxygen in your blood, reducing the oxygen supply to the fetus. Ultrasonic monitoring has shown reduced fetal movement after the mother smokes two cigarettes successively.

Secondary Smoke

If you are continually breathing in other people's smoke, your heartbeat and blood pressure may go up as you inhale smoke-filled air. If you don't have ashtrays out at home, even when you give a party, most guests will assume that your home is a smoke-free zone. We commonly see "no smoking" signs on doorways of homes and in many public places. Many offices do not permit smoking.

If you're timid about asking someone to put out a cigarette, do what a friend of ours does. She tells annoying smokers that she is pregnant and the smoke is making her sick to her stomach. Cigarettes are promptly extinguished.

Warning Labels

If you choose to smoke you probably choose to disregard the surgeon general's warning on the cigarette packages, ads, and billboards. When your action is potentially harmful to the child you're carrying, it's harder to ignore those warnings. Some women are highly motivated to give up smoking during pregnancy, but if you find you can't stop, you need special counseling. There are a number of stop-smoking programs especially geared to pregnant women.

Stopping smoking, even for the last few months of pregnancy, will improve your baby's potential growth and development. Cut back if you can't stop altogether. Make every effort to eat a balanced diet and gain adequate weight. Several reports suggest that greater prenatal weight gain helps offset the low birth weight of infants born to women who smoke (202). Your doctor may prescribe a vitamin-mineral supplement—but diet and supplements will not neutralize carbon monoxide, nicotine, and cyanides.

DRUGS: TAKING THEM AND DOING THEM

In the Medicine Cabinet

Drugs are chemicals that help with the diagnosis, cure, prevention, or treatment of an illness. But what is given to heal sometimes proves to be a hazard. Some years ago, women who took thalidomide, an apparently harmless tranquilizer used as a sleeping pill, produced malformed babies. The daughters of women who took a hormone called DES to prevent miscarriage have a greater incidence of cancer of the vagina and cervix.

More recently, isotretinoin, a concentrated form of vitamin A used to treat severe acne, has caused birth defects—after being used despite warnings on the label and letters to physicians. Since this drug is used primarily by women of childbearing age, the FDA and the manufacturer issued guidelines that the drug should always be used with an effective form of contraception (195).

The FDA requires extensive testing of drugs for potential hazards; many drugs contain warnings concerning use during pregnancy. Physicians avoid prescribing medications during pregnancy, if at all possible.

Retin-A, another vitamin A–derived drug, is not as dangerous as isotretinoin during pregnancy because it is used topically and little is absorbed into the body. But Retin-A should be used during pregnancy *only* if there is a very good reason for doing so (82). Prevention of signs of skin aging, a common use for Retin-A, isn't a good enough reason.

You should not be afraid to take medications if they are needed and prescribed by your doctor; both you and your baby must be kept healthy. The doctor has information about medications that have been proved safe or unsafe in pregnancy and lactation. *Never take any over-the-counter medication without first consulting your doctor.* Even the innocent cold tablets or aspirin can have negative effects. In aspirin, for example, the salicylate crosses the placenta freely and can be found in the fetal bloodstream at birth. Research indicates that aspirin may interfere with the development of normal circulation in the fetus and newborn, increase the risk of hemorrhage to the mother and newborn, and delay the onset of labor and extend its duration (177).

The Advisory Panel on Over-the-Counter Analgesics has recommended that women be warned not to take aspirin during the last three months of pregnancy unless under the advice and supervision of a physician (177).

If you have a condition that requires regularly prescribed medication, discuss the implications with your doctor or a specialist prior to becoming pregnant. Double-check medications prescribed by specialists with your obstetrician. It's better to ask too many questions than too few. If you take birth-control pills, stop using them at least three months before you attempt to conceive. If you become pregnant—or even think you are pregnant—while taking oral contraceptives, consult your doctor. If pregnancy is confirmed, stop taking them immediately.

Uppers and Downers

Amphetamines, barbiturates, and *tranquilizers* cross the placenta, thereby presenting a risk to the fetus. Both barbiturates and tranquilizers can create a fetal dependency on the drug, and drug-dependent newborns suffer withdrawal symptoms. Babies addicted to barbiturates display tremors, restlessness, and irritability. There is also evidence that use of tranquilizers early in pregnancy increases the risk of birth defects including cleft lip and palate (164). Like tranquilizers, amphetamines have been reported to cause birth defects. Years ago these drugs were commonly prescribed during pregnancy, but today most doctors no longer prescribe them for pregnant women unless they are necessary for the control of seizures or for psychiatric reasons.

Information on drug use during pregnancy remains fragmentary since ethical considerations rule out experiments on humans, and the results of experiments on animals may not be transferable to humans. The bottom line is that it's safest to be drug free. If you take amphetamines, barbiturates, or tranquilizers, give them up before you become pregnant. If you are already pregnant, seek the advice of someone who can help you stop.

"Social" Drugs

Marijuana use remains popular among women during their childbearing years. The extent of use during pregnancy isn't known, but it is estimated that 10 percent to 22 percent of pregnant women smoke pot at least occasionally (64). Marijuana is rapidly absorbed from the lungs into the bloodstream, where it is then processed by many tissues and by the liver. Marijuana alters many biological systems. Its active ingredients are stored in fat deposits and are excreted over time. It takes a week or more after smoking one joint for the residue to completely clear the body.

Like tobacco, marijuana increases heart rate and blood pressure, which may lead to reduced maternal blood flow into the placenta (60).

Marijuana use during pregnancy has been the subject of a number of studies in recent years. These studies have shown a variety of effects: reduced birth weight and body length, increased frequency of premature delivery, higher rates of premature labor, facial features similar to those induced by fetal alcohol syndrome, and altered neurologic responses at birth (172). The active ingredient of marijuana, tetrahydrocannabinol (THC), has been shown to have long-term effects on learning behavior in offspring of users (48).

What is clear is that marijuana may interfere with prenatal growth and development. It is dangerous for your baby.

Cocaine

During the 1980s, *cocaine* use grew to epidemic proportions. The National Institute on Drug Abuse estimates that ten out of every one hundred pregnant women have used or are using cocaine (98). One study of women from a poor urban area found that 18 percent had used cocaine at least once during pregnancy (205). Unlike some other drugs, cocaine is used by many financially privileged women; it is a drug that cuts across socioeconomic class lines.

Cocaine readily crosses the placenta, where it causes blood vessels to constrict, restricting nutrient flow and inhibiting growth of the fetus (172). It also increases heart rate and blood pressure (198). Because cocaine suppresses appetite (and diverts grocery money to supply the drug), the mother may further deprive the fetus with her irregular and inadequate eating habits.

Women who use cocaine are likely to have premature separation of the placenta and spontaneous abortion after intravenous injection or nasal use of the drug (29). If their babies do survive, they may be born prematurely, and tend to be in the low range for weight, length, and head circumference (75).

Women who fear that their drug use will be detected from urine analysis may avoid prenatal medical care, increasing the risks to the unborn child even more. If using drugs is keeping you from getting proper care, talk with a drug counselor who can help you find an understanding and knowledgeable physician who can provide medical and nutritional support.

Narcotics and Hallucinogens

Attaining euphoria is the goal of those who take *narcotic analgesics*. This category of drugs includes heroin, morphine, codeine, oxycodone (Percodan), Demerol, and methadone. While there are many differences in sources and processing, all of these drugs are addictive to both mother and baby. As a side effect, narcotics cause appetite loss, making maintaining good nutritional status difficult.

Psychedelic drugs achieved great popularity in the 1960s, but have been used since ancient times. While older psychedelic drugs were derived from seeds and other parts of plants, new drugs are developed in chemical laboratories. Many people who use hallucinogens also abuse other drugs, particularly stimulants such as amphetamines.

LSD is a potent hallucinogen that arouses the central nervous system. It is a chemically modified ergot alkaloid. Like other ergots, it causes uterine contractions and is suspected of causing fetal damage and death.

PCP is a street drug that is a potent hallucinogen, acting as both a central nervous system stimulant and depressant. It produces severe psychiatric reactions similar to schizophrenia. The impaired judgment and abuse to the body caused by PCP jeopardizes both mother and baby.

Potentially harmful substance use and abuse during pregnancy has long-term implications: babies born with mental and physical retardation that lasts a lifetime—yours and theirs.

8

Special Needs of Pregnancy

There is nothing very beautiful or fulfilling about morning sickness—or hemorrhoids, constipation, and swollen ankles, for that matter. But considering all the changes that take place in your body during pregnancy, it's understandable that many women might experience discomfort and occasional complications. If you know why a particular physical reaction occurs and know what to do about it, you may be less concerned if it happens to you. The reactions we address in this chapter are those related to your diet.

COMMON PROBLEMS

Nausea and Vomiting

Anne was one of those women who believed that morning sickness was all psychological. She was never sick a day during any of her three pregnancies. Only after spending time with a newly pregnant friend who was experiencing her sixth consecutive day of vomiting did she believe that morning sickness was not "all in the head"! More than half of all pregnant women experience morning sickness, and it is physically very real (194).

Morning sickness usually begins about six weeks after the start of the last menstrual period. It is most common in first pregnancies. For women who have irregular menstrual periods, it's often the first sign of pregnancy. Mary, who had been told that she could not have children, got a "flu" while traveling in Europe that made her sick, tired, and irritable. She thought it was related to the water and not sleeping well at night. A friend advised her to have a pregnancy test as soon as she got home, and when the test came back positive, Mary didn't know who was more shocked, her husband, her doctor, or herself!

JeanMarie Brownson, test-kitchen director of the Chicago *Tribune,* blamed her *mal de mere* on the rich foods she ate in her job as a restaurant critic. On a family camping trip, JeanMarie and her pregnant sister-in-law found themselves side by side in the bathroom each morning, suffering from very similar upsets. The food expert had misdiagnosed her symptoms!

If you consider pregnancy a possibility, you're more likely to be aware of the first subtle signs of conception. For others, like Mary and JeanMarie, persistent nausea is a signal that cannot be dismissed. It's hard to think of morning sickness as positive. But it does make you pay attention to what is happening, and it can alert you to take care during the early critical stages of fetal growth and development.

The not-so-wonderful thing about morning sickness is that although it usually occurs in the morning, you can experience it any time of the day or night—or on occasion, for a whole day or night. It generally disappears about the fourteenth week of pregnancy, but don't be surprised if you are still nauseated on day one hundred.

CAUSES

Since morning sickness is considered a "mild" problem and the affliction disappears of its own accord within weeks, little research has been conducted to discover its cause or to develop therapies. The most popular theory is that morning sickness is brought on by changing hormone levels. HCG, the hormone that indicates pregnancy in urine and blood tests, is at high levels during the first trimester. As it decreases, so does nausea (52). Another theory suggests that morning sickness is caused by increased estrogen production (202).

Yet another explanation is that nausea is caused when cells of the fertilized ovum invade the endometrium and begin rapid division. Degenerative by-products, similar to those produced by radiation or burn therapy, may cause nausea and vomiting (202).

For some women, emotional factors contribute to nausea or vomiting. Morning sickness is unknown in some very simple societies with low levels of stress; pregnant women hospitalized for nausea often have none in the more tranquil hospital environment; women with wanted pregnancies tend to have less morning sickness than those with unplanned pregnancies. Some women experience great anxiety and stress when they find they are pregnant. This can interfere with digestion and cause nausea all by itself.

Nausea is not pleasant, but most will agree that vomiting is worse. The real danger in vomiting is that reduced food intake and a loss of fluids can lead to weakness and dehydration. Often nausea can be controlled so that vomiting doesn't occur. Curiously, several studies show that morning sickness is associated with *favorable* pregnancy outcomes (179).

TREATMENT

The traditional advice to nauseated pregnant women is to eat crackers. A friend of ours says, "I've never eaten so many crackers in my life as I did during my first three months of pregnancy! I still feel nauseated when I see a box of saltines."

Medical journals document both the frustrations and the creative treatments of physicians who have tried to alleviate the discomforts of morning sickness. In the first century, the Roman physician Soranus recommended hitting a leather bag, and if that didn't do it, a woman was to be bound and immersed in hot water (59).

At one time, severe nausea was routinely treated with a drug called Bendectin. Despite the extensive testing and safe use of the drug by more than thirty million women, there were a number of lawsuits claiming that Bendectin was the cause of birth defects. Bendectin was voluntarily removed from the market by the manufacturer in June 1983.

Vitamin B_6 has also been used to treat nausea and vomiting during pregnancy. Injections or oral doses ranging from ten to one hundred milligrams have brought relief to some women. In 1979, the American Medical Association Council on Drugs found that there was no scientific evidence that the vitamin is effective in treating nausea. A recent review of safety and efficacy of drug treatment of nausea during pregnancy supports the AMA council's position (109). Rather than taking a supplement, include foods that are rich in vitamin B_6 in your diet. Taking one of the B vitamins alone can upset the balance and utilization of other vitamins and should only be done under medical supervision.

WHAT TO DO IF YOU ARE NAUSEATED

- Eat frequent, small meals—as often as every two hours.
- Keep your carbohydrate level up. Carbs are easy to digest, provide energy, and free up protein for fetal growth.
- Avoid high-fat and rich foods.
- Eat a high-protein snack before you go to bed.
- Keep crackers, popcorn, dry cereal, or vanilla wafers next to your bed. Eat something when you wake up but before you get up. Doing so will start the digestive process that will remove excess acid from your stomach and relieve nausea. Have your breakfast after the nausea subsides.
- Get up slowly—sudden movement can aggravate nausea.
- Be sure you have fresh air in the room where you sleep.
- Avoid cooking odors; let your partner fix his own and the family's breakfast.
- If you're taking iron supplements, take them an hour before or two hours after a meal, with a liquid such as water or orange juice (202). Or ask your doctor if you can delay taking the supplements for a few weeks until the nausea passes.
- Do not drink beverages or soup with meals, but be sure to get enough liquids between meals, especially if you are vomiting. Fruit juice and carbonated beverages are easy to digest and will supply some needed carbohydrates if you are having difficulty keeping down foods.
- What makes one woman sick is soothing to another woman. Foods commonly experienced as either very good or very bad are milk and tea. Most women find cold foods and beverages easier to take than hot ones. Curiously, some women enjoy spicy foods like pizza even when they're nauseated (158).

- Stop smoking. Smoking increases secretion of stomach acid, which can cause nausea.
- Listen to your body and do whatever seems to work for you

It's very unlikely that severe morning sickness will cause you to lose your baby. And vomiting in early pregnancy will not have a negative effect on the birth weight of your baby (52). If you are nauseated often, have a poor appetite, and can't keep down what you do eat, try to eat whenever you can. Drink enough fluids to avoid getting dehydrated. Small high-carbohydrate meals, eaten at regular intervals, will provide a steady source of calories and will prevent your body from burning fat stores. Eat what you can, even if that means nothing but ginger ale, popsicles, and hard candy—your digestive system is very resourceful about capturing calories (158). Some women manage to keep food down when they eat immediately after vomiting. Try not to allow yourself to get hungry. By keeping something in your stomach you may be able to avoid nausea.

About 2 percent of pregnant women have sustained and prolonged nausea and vomiting. This condition is quite rare but can become very dangerous. Its technical name is *hyper-*

Inform your doctor if

- You are vomiting and unable to keep down fluids
- You vomit more than twice a day
- You are still nauseated and vomiting after your fourteenth week of pregnancy
- You are losing weight

emesis gravidarum. If it continues, dehydration, acidosis, severe fluid and electrolyte imbalance, and weight loss can occur. The condition is more common among women who have had anorexia nervosa or bulimia before pregnancy. Hospitalization may be required.

Increased Appetite and Cravings

Pregnancy is a time when most women experience an increase in appetite. In addition, cravings and aversions are more likely to occur during pregnancy than at any other time in life (172). In one study of 463 women who had recently delivered babies, more than 90 percent reported a craving for at least one food item during the last trimester of pregnancy, and more than 50 percent said they had an aversion to at least one food (201).

CAUSES

At about the twelfth week of pregnancy your appetite may begin to increase. This increase cannot be attributed to a higher need for calories at this stage of pregnancy; a battle of hormones is to blame. During the first half of pregnancy, more of the hormone progesterone, an appetite stimulant, is produced than estrogen, an appetite depressant (197). Estrogen increases as pregnancy progresses, and some women find that their appetite wanes as they approach delivery. Other studies show appetite decreasing during the first trimester, improving in the fifth month, and then waning as delivery approaches (12).

Some pregnant women have a metallic taste in their mouth that changes their sense of taste. Coffee and tea may no longer taste good, for instance. You may crave more salt, suggesting that there is a connection between taste and physiological need (21). Cravings for ice and nonfood items (see page 176) may be related to iron needs.

TREATMENT

Satisfy your increased appetite with more nutritious food, not just more of any food. Go ahead and indulge your food cravings, as long as they don't keep you from eating a variety of nutritious foods.

Tell your doctor if you crave something unusual, especially if it isn't a normal food item—it may be an indication that you need more iron. Your doctor may want to check for other problems as well.

Constipation and Frequent Urination

Everyday toilet routines are an important part of your life when you are pregnant! Many of the bowel and bladder problems of pregnancy can be solved by simple dietary changes. Avoid the over-the-counter remedies you may have used before pregnancy.

CAUSES

Two factors impair bowel and bladder functioning when you are pregnant. First, the uterus grows and puts pressure on your bladder and intestines. Second, hormones of pregnancy slow the muscle action of the intestines.

A frequent need to urinate is not surprising, considering that your bladder is being pushed, kicked, and shoved. It is also being pressed into ever-tighter quarters by your growing uterus. The expansion of the uterus begins early in pregnancy, causing the sensation of a full bladder—one of the early signs of pregnancy. As food passes more slowly through the stomach and intestines, maximum amounts of nutrients and fluids are extracted. The food mass is moved along slowly by smooth muscles that have been relaxed by hormones produced from the beginning of pregnancy. Your kidneys are also working harder to deal with the increase in blood and body fluids that are necessary for your pregnancy. The result can be irregularity, constipation, and maybe hemorrhoids.

TREATMENT

There are several things you can do to alleviate these problems. For one, get some *exercise* each day. Several exercises taught at Lamaze and other childbirth classes may improve the muscle tone of the bladder. Exercise also helps to keep things moving along if you're constipated. Other measures you may take—

- Empty your bladder frequently.
- To avoid "leaking," do exercises, such as the Kegel exercise, to strengthen your pelvic floor muscles. The Kegel exercise is done by tightening and then relaxing the muscles that you use when urinating. You can practice while you drive, sit at a desk, or watch television.
- Constipation can be reduced by drinking plenty of liquids—at least eight glasses of water a day.
- Eat high-fiber foods (dried and fresh fruits, bran cereals, whole grains, raw vegetables) that help hold water in the stool.
- Eat prunes or figs or drink prune juice. These fruits contain isatin, a natural laxative.

If you do become constipated, *do not take laxatives* unless they are prescribed by your doctor. Mineral oil inhibits vitamin and mineral absorption and should be avoided. Your doctor may prescribe a stool softener instead of a laxative. Or try one of the old-fashioned remedies that still work: a glass of warm water with lemon juice in it, prunes, or prune juice. Iron supplements can be constipating. Your doctor may make an adjustment in your supplement prescription if iron is aggravating the situation.

Many women need rest room pit stops midmeal, after a meal, and then an hour later. Nothing really can be done about this. Drinking less fluid during the late evening hours may allow you to sleep through at least half the night. When you are resting, especially at the later stages of pregnancy, lie on your side so that the uterus is not pressing on blood vessels to the kidneys, inhibiting them from working properly.

Hemorrhoids

Hemorrhoids are a form of varicose veins that swell in small round lumps in or around the anus. Many women experience hemorrhoids during pregnancy.

CAUSES

The increased size of the uterus puts pressure on the veins in your rectum. They sometimes protrude in and around the anus, causing burning and itching. Occasionally, hemorrhoids may rupture and bleed.

TREATMENT

Treatment involves relieving pressure and soothing the pain and itching.

- Avoid constipation. Drink lots of water and eat more fruits and vegetables and fiber foods.
- Avoid straining during elimination.
- Get an inflatable ring to sit on. Covering it like a seat cushion may make it more presentable at work!
- Apply ice packs or take warm (not hot) baths. Both can provide relief.
- Relieve itching and burning with topical ointments such as petroleum jelly, or ask your doctor to recommend a safe suppository.
- Lie down at various times during the day to relieve pressure caused by the uterus pushing down on the lower intestine.

Heartburn

Heartburn is not related to your heart but is a burning sensation in the lower esophagus, close to your heart. Sometimes it feels as if you've eaten too much and you're uncomfortably full.

CAUSES

Heartburn typically occurs during the last three months of pregnancy when your baby is growing and pushing on the surrounding organs. As food follows its normal downward route, the expanding uterus compresses the stomach; digested food and stomach fluids are pushed back into your esophagus. During pregnancy, the valve between the esophagus and the stomach is more relaxed than usual, so food can easily reverse direction. The sour taste accompanying heartburn comes from stomach acids that rise to your throat.

TREATMENT

Heartburn can be relieved with antacids, but many antacids interfere with absorption of important vitamins and minerals. Constant neutralization of acid makes it difficult to absorb iron. Ask your doctor to prescribe a suitable medication. Do not take medications containing sodium bicarbonate (baking soda) or large amounts of sodium, such as Alka-Seltzer, that can promote fluid retention above and beyond what you need for pregnancy. It makes more sense to reduce the discomforts of heartburn through dietary control and by putting your body in a comfortable position.

- Relax and eat slowly.
- Rather than three large meals, eat small meals at frequent intervals.
- Limit fluids at meals.
- Stimulate salivation by chewing gum or sucking on a sour lemon drop. Saliva is naturally alkaline and may help neutralize acid in the esophagus (81).
- If a specific food bothers you, avoid it. Common heartburners: Mexican and Italian food; fast-food hamburgers; coffee, tea, colas (decaf varieties don't help); spicy or high-fat foods; tomato products; citrus fruits and juices; chocolate and after-dinner mints (81).
- Wear comfortable, loose-fitting clothes.
- Stop smoking (yet another reason).
- Wait several hours after eating to exercise.
- Do not bend over or lie down flat after you eat. Use an extra pillow. Raise the top of your bed six inches by placing blocks or books under the legs of the bed.
- Walk around to encourage gastric juices to flow down, not up.

- Never take antacids without your doctor's specific direction to do so.

Aches, Pains, and Cramps

All sorts of little pains, and sometimes not-so-little pains, occur especially during the last weeks of pregnancy. Muscle cramps in the legs and abdomen are frequent, especially at night when you are tired. Sometimes a fetus feels as if it's doing calisthenics in the womb, constantly kicking the mother.

CAUSES

Most pains are caused by poor circulation and pressure of the growing baby on your stomach, bladder, nerves, intestines, ribs, lungs, and what sometimes seems like every muscle and bone in your body. Pain in the pubic area and around your thighs is caused by the baby pressing on nerves, or by pelvic joints softening in preparation for labor.

TREATMENT

One school of thought says that cramps are caused by a calcium deficiency and recommends *increasing* dairy products or taking calcium supplements. Another school attributes cramps to an imbalance of calcium and phosphorus, and advocates *reducing* milk, which is high in both minerals. Studies do not support these therapies (77; 173).

For some women, wearing support hose during the day and alternating periods of rest and activity helps eliminate leg cramps (47). Elevating your legs or pressing your foot against a hard surface may bring some relief. Rapid, firm massaging while moving your foot up and down will reduce a cramp, but it may continue to hurt for some time. Take a short walk or do exercises to stretch your calf muscles before you go to bed.

If pain is severe or prolonged, call your doctor. This is true of any pain. Prolonged pain may be caused by a blood clot, although this is rare.

Edema

Edema (swelling, particularly of the hands and feet) during the last trimester of pregnancy is normal and should not be confused with the kind of edema that accompanies nonpregnant conditions. If accompanied by high blood pressure, protein in your urine, nausea, and other symptoms, edema may be an indication of preeclampsia (discussed later in this chapter). For most women, however, edema is part of normal pregnancy. In fact, some edema during pregnancy is beneficial (128); women who have mild edema have slightly larger babies and a lower rate of prematurity (202).

CAUSES

Estrogen, the same hormone that causes some women to retain water in their bodies just before they menstruate, causes water retention during pregnancy. Connective tissues become more elastic during the last months of pregnancy. These softer tissues dilate more easily during labor and delivery. Estrogen in the tissues attracts and holds water. "Reservoirs" form in your ankles, hands, and legs; some women feel as if their whole body is puffy. These water-filled cells help hold your expanded blood volume during pregnancy, offset losses that occur during delivery, and contribute to the production of breast milk. Meanwhile, you will probably be more comfortable if you buy a pair of shoes a size bigger than usual!

Most of this fluid is lost during delivery, but some edema may remain after the baby is born. The remaining fluid is usually excreted during the week after delivery as your hormonal balance shifts (5; 8).

TREATMENT

Salt restriction and diuretics (water pills) are no longer routinely advised to relieve edema. The additional fluid in your body when you're pregnant actually *increases* your need for sodium. If sodium is restricted, your body has to work harder to control the movement of fluids in and out of cells. Diuretics remove fluids and sodium by increasing urination. Use of diuretics can cause nausea, vomiting, headache, and loss of appetite. They should be used only in special situations determined by your doctor.

Edema should be monitored by your doctor to make sure that it is not accompanied by other symptoms. But if you have "normal" edema, the following will bring relief:

- Since swelling in your legs and feet is aggravated by the pressure of the uterus as it presses on your veins, rest on your left side with a pillow under your feet four or five times a day. This position permits better return circulation of blood from your legs.
- Wear comfortable shoes that allow your feet to expand.
- Remove tight rings.
- Lie on your side to allow the kidneys to work more efficiently when you sleep. Some excess water may be

held in tissues because the growing baby is blocking normal flow to the kidneys.
- Do not take diuretics or limit salt.

BEYOND SELF-HELP

Up to this point, the problems described, if not abnormally severe, can be treated by modifying your diet, exercising, or trying relief methods that you can manage on your own. Of course, you will want to tell your doctor, but generally you can manage the control measures.

Some nutrition-related complications during pregnancy, however, require careful medical monitoring and supervision, and dietary modification beyond the scope of this book—perhaps beyond the care that can be given by your regular physician.

If you encounter complications such as those described in the following pages, you will want to seek information about current treatments, specialists, and facilities available in your area. We offer some explanation only so that you will know what to expect.

Anemia

One problem with anemia is that many women think they have it when they don't, while other women don't think they have it when they do. You are not anemic just because you feel tired. *Anemia* occurs when hemoglobin levels fall far below the average for healthy women of the same age and stage of pregnancy (172). The only way to know if you are anemic is to have a blood test, which is routinely done early in pregnancy. Another test for anemia is usually done at your six-week exam after delivering.

CAUSES

Nutrition-based anemia during pregnancy and the postnatal period is most likely to be caused by iron depletion. Low folate and B_{12} intakes may cause other types of anemia.

Women of childbearing age are at risk for developing iron deficiency anemia because many have poor iron stores and cannot meet the high demands for iron imposed during pregnancy. Iron deficiency anemia is a common nutritional problem for American women. At the beginning of the second trimester, your needs for iron and folate increase dramatically. Your expanded blood volume requires iron; rapid fetal cell division and growth increases your need for folate. Pregnant women, especially women carrying more than one fetus, are most at risk for developing folate and vitamin B_{12} anemias.

During the third trimester, your baby builds up reserves of iron that will last for the first few months of life. The baby takes what it needs from the mother; few babies are born with poor iron reserves (172).

It may take as long as two years for a woman to recover the iron lost during pregnancy and delivery (202). As many as 30 percent of new mothers may have folate deficiencies nine weeks after giving birth (138).

TREATMENT

If you suspect you're anemic, see your doctor about a blood test. The doctor will determine appropriate treatment if you need it. To ensure you get enough iron:

- Pay special attention to your diet before conception
- Eat foods rich in iron, folate, and vitamin B_{12}
- Take supplements, if prescribed, according to directions
- Build up iron and folate reserves between pregnancies

Diabetes Mellitus

Not too many years ago, women with diabetes or other chronic diseases were advised not to have children. Now many of these women can and do have healthy babies. Closely monitored pregnancies of women with diabetes are 95 percent successful today (7). But it requires extra care and commitment, both physically and emotionally. The advances of modern science make possible many babies that are truly miracles.

Diabetes is a disorder that occurs when the pancreas produces insufficient or ineffective insulin. Insulin is needed to turn carbohydrate from food into energy. Without insulin, blood sugar (glucose) from carbohydrate breakdown is trapped in the bloodstream.

Hunger is an early sign of diabetes because glucose doesn't enter the cells of the brain. Thirst is another symptom because the kidneys want to get rid of excess blood sugar that spills into the urine.

Some diabetes can be treated with diet, but some people can control diabetes only through supplemental insulin therapy.

Two types of diabetes occur during pregnancy: diabetes that existed before pregnancy and will remain after delivery; and diabetes that begins during pregnancy and disappears after birth.

PREEXISTING DIABETES

Most women with this form of diabetes know they have it, have been treating it with insulin and/or diet, and will continue to have it after delivery. If you have this type of diabetes, discuss the implications of pregnancy with your doctor before you stop birth-control measures and attempt to become pregnant (69). Being in good metabolic control before conception and in the early weeks of pregnancy reduces the incidence of birth defects and lowers risk in general. During the early weeks of pregnancy, fetal organs are forming (70). Dr. Myron Winick believes that vitamin-mineral supplements should be given to all women with diabetes who plan to become pregnant and that they should be continued throughout all high-risk pregnancies (197).

The physician who helps you manage your diabetes may recommend an obstetrician who will treat you during your pregnancy or with whom he or she can work to supervise your care. The specific plan of care will be based on the duration of your diabetes, existing complications, and your physical and emotional needs. Most women with diabetes mellitus are on insulin therapy during pregnancy. The insulin may be different from the type you have used before and you may have to inject it several times a day to regulate your blood sugar levels. Some women use an insulin pump that releases insulin when blood sugar levels get too high.

Your diet and medications will have to be changed throughout your pregnancy as your hormonal levels shift and the baby grows. Expect to strictly control your food intake and the sugar levels in your blood and urine. You may be hospitalized for blood-sugar monitoring at the beginning and at times during your pregnancy.

Babies born to women with diabetes tend to be larger than

babies born to women without diabetes. Frequently these babies are delivered several weeks early to permit normal vaginal delivery. This can often be controlled by good diabetes management. Babies born to mothers who have diabetes are carefully monitored the first few days after birth until their hormonal regulation is well established. If you want to breast-feed, you can, but you will need guidance from a registered dietitian, registered nurse, or your physician.

IF YOU HAVE DIABETES

- Your baby will have the very best chance if you keep your blood glucose as close to normal as possible during your entire pregnancy. A controlled diet is essential to the management of diabetes and can reduce the incidence and severity of many of its symptoms and complications. A diet will be devised just for you based on your specific habits and needs. Although almost all of the information in this book is applicable, the specific number of servings and types of food must be modified to meet your individual needs, with frequent reassessments as the pregnancy progresses. You may be told to work with a registered dietitian or certified diabetes educator who can counsel you about your diet.
- Several complications of pregnancy are more common in women who have diabetes. These include pregnancy-induced hypertension (discussed later in this chapter), excessive fluid surrounding the baby, and prematurity. Complications of diabetes are sometimes intensified during pregnancy, such as changes in the retina of the eye and in the kidneys (150).
- Diabetes is a high-risk situation in pregnancy. Care of a pregnant woman with diabetes requires full knowledge of the altered me-

tabolism of both pregnancy and diabetes. It can be very tricky and requires strict medical management. Very high or very low blood sugar levels can be dangerous to your baby and to you. You will be instructed to test your blood sugar level often and make dietary or insulin adjustments to keep your blood sugar within a specific range.

- Your doctor can often detect early signs of problems or potential complications. Find a good doctor whom you like because you will see him or her often.
- Ultrasound monitoring is likely to be done at regular intervals throughout your pregnancy. Ultrasound shows growth and development of your baby and detects problems very early, should they occur (143).

If you have diabetes and are considering having a baby or are already pregnant, there are many resources for you. Call your local affiliate chapter of the American Diabetes Association and ask for the information they have on diabetes in pregnancy. One of their publications, *Diabetes Forecast,* has a number of excellent articles on the subject.

GESTATIONAL DIABETES

During the second half of pregnancy, hormones are produced by the placenta that oppose the action of insulin. This situation creates an extra demand on the pancreas to produce more insulin. If it cannot, *gestational diabetes,* which begins during pregnancy and disappears after delivery, occurs.

From 2 to 3 percent of all pregnant women—sixty thousand to one hundred thousand women each year in the United States—develop diabetes during their pregnancies. Some expert groups recommend screening all pregnant women with a blood sugar test between the twenty-fourth and twenty-eighth weeks of pregnancy, even if there are no apparent symptoms (69). Gestational diabetes usually occurs during the latter half of pregnancy when there is an increased need for insulin. It disappears after the baby's birth, although many women affected develop diabetes later in life. Avoiding obesity is recommended to reduce the risk of diabetes after pregnancy.

If tests for levels of sugar in the blood or urine show that you have gestational diabetes, your obstetrician may recommend that you be evaluated by an internist, diabetologist, or endocrinologist. All of these medical specialists have additional training in the management of pregnant women with diabetes. Some obstetricians prefer to manage the gestational diabetic more directly, for this form of diabetes is usually less difficult to control and generally has fewer complications than insulin-dependent diabetes. Blood sugar levels, age, and other factors will determine whether you need daily insulin injections or can control the diabetes by diet alone (143).

Hypertension

Hypertension is the medical term for *high blood pressure.* Like sugar in your urine, high blood pressure is a sign that something is not working as it should. Because several types of hypertension can occur during pregnancy, your doctor will want to determine the reason before suggesting treatment.

Many women in this country, especially low-income women, experience hypertension during their childbearing years (202). Some are aware they have it before they become pregnant; others find out when their blood pressure is taken at the doctor's office. Some may develop hypertension as the result of problems directly related to pregnancy. Others have a temporary hypertension only during labor and immediately after birth—in this situation, blood pressure returns to normal within ten days.

Regardless of its cause, elevations in blood pressure must be treated to avoid endangering either mother or baby. Medications may be prescribed and rest will be absolutely essential, combined with careful medical monitoring.

Pregnancy-Induced Hypertension (PIH)

PIH was formerly called *toxemia.* Some doctors still use that term today, though strictly speaking it's a misnomer, deriving from *tox* (meaning poison) and *emia* (meaning of the blood). It was originally thought to be caused by water retention as a result of eating too much salt. Early treatment included fluid and salt restriction. This theory has been disproven. Instead, emphasis is now placed on increasing the quality of the total diet—not restricting it.

Pregnancy-induced hypertension can be prevented in many cases by good prenatal care and sound eating habits. Adequate calories are important to free up protein to do its job. Protein and minerals help maintain fluid and electrolyte status, blood volume, and tissue growth. Vitamins are necessary for growth and proper metabolism.

In addition to poor diet, both before and during pregnancy, statistics point toward other risk factors. Women who are most likely to develop PIH are those who

- Have mothers or sisters who developed PIH during their first pregnancies

- Are in their first pregnancy; PIH is less common in later pregnancies
- Are carrying more than one baby
- Are in their first pregnancy and are less than twenty years old or are thirty-five years or older
- Have existing high blood pressure, kidney disease, diabetes, or inadequate medical care (168)

It is generally agreed that weight gain of more than thirty pounds is *not* a factor. This figure, which was once believed to be the most weight that a woman could safely gain, is now considered well within normal limits. In fact, early work by Dr. Winslow T. Tompkins, a pioneer in research on maternal nutritional status in the first half of this century, found an increased incidence of PIH among women who were *underweight* at conception and failed to gain enough weight during their pregnancy (181). Thus, part of the dilemma of PIH may be the duration of poor nutritional status as well as actual food consumed during pregnancy.

Among several disorders associated with PIH are *preeclampsia, severe preeclampsia,* and *eclampsia.* Preeclampsia is described as a general edema including fluid retention in the hands and face, high blood pressure (hypertension), and protein in the urine. A weight gain of over two pounds (verified on your doctor's scale) in one week is an indication of potential preeclampsia in the last trimester. Bed rest, a good diet, and medical care may arrest the situation, but hospitalization may be necessary. In preeclampsia, there is a significant decrease in blood flow to the placenta.

Severe preeclampsia is a more acute form of eclampsia that occurs when blood pressure and other symptoms increase in degree. Danger signs are blurred vision, headache, or abdominal pain. If any of these signs occur, call your doctor immediately. Both you and your baby are in extreme danger if it is truly eclampsia.

If preeclampsia goes untreated, convulsions and coma may occur. This is eclampsia—a life-threatening condition! But don't panic if you have a headache—it may be just that.

PIH during pregnancy remains the subject of much speculation and medical debate. Recent studies suggest that increasing calcium can reduce PIH and preeclampsia, but this is not conclusive (13). It may be that preeclampsia is related to antibody reactions between maternal and fetal tissues (151).

We wish we could say that if you eat a balanced diet, you will not get pregnancy-induced hypertension. Unfortunately, we cannot.

If you are eating a nutritious diet, following the advice in this book, and getting good prenatal care, you are doing everything we know of at this time to prevent PIH.

Heart and Kidney Disease

Pregnancy makes increased demands if a woman's heart or kidneys are not functioning normally. Heart disease is the one situation in which a low-sodium diet plays a major role in medical management of pregnancy. Your care must be closely supervised by medical specialists. Rest and dietary modifications will surely be parts of the plan, customized for your individual physiological problems.

Other medical problems can occur during pregnancy, but this book deals only with those conditions in which nutrition is a factor. We do not want to minimize the necessity for care in other situations, and we advise you always to get medical advice from your physician.

9

The Feeding Track: Breast or Bottle?

Before your baby is born, you need to think about whether to breast-feed or bottle-feed. Now is the time to gather information, evaluate your situation in relation to home and work, talk with those who are close to you, and make a decision. Your decision may influence your choice of physician, types of medication used during delivery, and even hospital. If you expect to return to work, it will certainly influence those plans. Indecision or disagreements about feeding during the emotionally fragile days following delivery can be upsetting. Regardless of how you choose to feed your baby, you will need to know what to expect so you can make the necessary preparations.

This chapter will *not* tell you how to make formula or stimulate the let-down reflex to initiate nursing. That information is available from other sources. This book deals with your pregnancy and decisions and actions during this time, not after your baby is born.

You may already be pretty sure about how you want to feed your baby, but please don't close the book. Reading this chapter can support the decision you have already made by pointing out advantages. It may bring up situations that you hadn't thought about but that deserve consideration. Or it may open up new ways of looking at feeding that will change your mind. Whatever your thoughts, you will feel better about your decision if you examine the pros and cons of both breast- and bottle-feeding, and choose what is right for you.

RECOMMENDATIONS AND REALITIES

Hormonally and metabolically, pregnancy does not stop when the baby is born. The minute the placenta is expelled, the lactation process begins. Lactation is a function of the pregnancy state. Even the makers of infant formula concede that "breast is best." The health goals of the nation call for more and longer breast-feeding of our babies (176). The American Academy of Pediatrics, the American Medical Association, the American Public Health Association, and the American Dietetic Association all endorse breast-feeding as the preferred method of infant feeding. All over the world, nutrition-conscious professionals are committed to breast-feeding as a way to improve the health of future generations.

Then why is breast-feeding not the primary way to feed infants in this country? In 1987, 55 percent of new mothers were nursing when they left the hospital; by 1990, that number had fallen to 50 percent and of those who did start nursing, only half were still doing it six weeks later (152;23).

"It's a matter of exposure," says Patricia L. Bull, R.N., who is a certified lactation consultant. Her comment has double meaning. Many of us have never been around women who have breast-fed and we know very little about it; we don't see women breast-feeding on television, in movies, or in advertisements. Some think of women who nurse their babies in public as being exhibitionists; some of us are uncomfortable seeing a woman breast-feed even if it's in her own home! Pat Bull was asked to remove a breast-feeding poster from the wall in her hospital office. For some, the message is that breast-feeding is outside the social norm or even indecent.

"The information on breast-feeding makes it sound very difficult," Bull concedes. "Women worry about having enough milk, about milk that's too weak, frequent feedings, engorged breasts, and going back to work." Many of these concerns and potential problems can be alleviated through education and preventive action. Dr. Ruth A. Lawrence, in her book, *Breastfeeding: A Guide for the Medical Profession,* summarizes the need for public education on the subject:

> Education to put breast-feeding in the mainstream and to classify it as normal behavior has to start with preschoolers and continue through the educational system. Courses in biology, nutrition, health, and human sexuality should all include the breast and its functions. Dolls should not come with bottles. The media should include breast-feeding, not always bottle-feeding, in reference to young infants. Public policy should facilitate breast-feeding and provide space in public buildings and in the work place (108).

Observations show that breast-fed babies are generally healthier during the first year of life. Human milk contains immunity carriers, antibodies, and infection fighters called macrophages that protect the infant's digestive tract from bacteria and allergies. Many of these "big macs" have only recently been discovered. Even if these macrophages could be replicated in prepared formula, they would be destroyed by heat during processing. "Taking it unpasteurized, directly from the breast, is a benefit formula can't duplicate," says dietitian Ellyn Satter (158).

Data from other countries and previous decades clearly show that bottle-fed babies have a higher rate of infant mortality than breast-fed babies, primarily from diarrhea and malnutrition. Where sanitation, a safe water supply, refrigeration, and money to buy formula are severely limited, bottle-feeding is clearly not a viable option. In our country, however, most babies can grow and thrive on either breast or bottle milk. There are definite differences, and if the decision about what to feed your baby were being made only on the basis of the nutritional composition of the milk and its immune properties, there would be little question as to your choice. The reality is that the decision is influenced by a number of other factors.

Many first-time mothers today have little idea what is involved in either breast- or bottle-feeding an infant. There was a time when most women of childbearing age had grown up in extended families where there were young babies, so they picked up a lot of know-how. Today's mother may have had little hands-on experience with babies. She may never have even seen a baby being nursed or prepared a bottle. She may not have any idea about what constitutes a normal feeding pattern.

This book will present you with new facts and undo myths and misunderstandings about *both* breast- and bottle-feeding. In our experience, there are as many who have closed minds and prejudiced attitudes about infant formula feeding as those who see breast-feeding as disgusting or "overly maternal." We hope that your decision on how to feed your baby will be made only after you have reviewed all the facts about both breast- and bottle-feeding in the light of what is right for you and your family. We do not want to make you feel guilty if you do not choose to breast-feed—if breast-feeding isn't right for you, then it isn't right for your child. *Good parenting is a great deal more important than the kind of milk you give your baby.*

WHAT'S IN MILK

Milk is a product of evolution, produced by mammals to nourish their offspring during the delicate period after leaving the womb. The same nutrients are present in milk of all mammals, but the composition of each is different. Mother's milk is designed to meet the specific needs of the species. The baby whale, for example, has enormous energy needs, but cannot stay under water for long periods of time to nurse. The mother whale's milk is very concentrated, and a little takes the baby a long way. Human babies, on the other hand, because they grow slowly (at least compared to whales), do not need great quantities of nutrients; they thrive on frequent, small feedings.

Both breast milk and infant formula can provide adequate calories for the first five to six months. Human milk is considered the perfect food for an infant's needs and digestive system.

Like any other food, milk can be broken down into its nutritional components: carbohydrate, fat, protein, vitamins, minerals, and water. Scientists can actually write a recipe, or formula, for human milk, listing the amount of each key ingredient. Though it cannot exactly replicate human milk, cow milk can be modified to meet the specifications by adding and subtracting various components. Some infant formulas now on the market have a base made from soybeans for those who are allergic to cow milk. Formulas are also available that are tailored to the needs of premature infants, infants who need extra calories, or those who have other special needs. Infant formulas are regulated by strict quality control procedures and all meet standards developed by the American Academy of Pediatrics (192).

The exact content of human milk varies from mother to mother, day to day, morning to night, first minute of feeding to last, from one meal the mother eats to the next. The composition of breast milk also changes over time to meet the needs of the baby. Many women are distressed when they see that the substance coming first from their breast is a yellowish transparent liquid that does not look at all like milk. This substance, which proceeds regular milk, is *colostrum*. The nursing baby receives colostrum during the first three to five days of life, until the milk comes in. Some women may find that the colostrum does not flow immediately, but only after the baby sucks at her breast. This is quite normal, and should not cause her to worry; even a little will meet the baby's needs.

With mature milk, at first the milk is low in fat, but as a feeding progresses, the fat level increases. The baby stops nursing and resumes sucking only when put to the other breast where the milk is again low in fat (158). Some expressed milk samples look like skim milk and others look like heavy cream with clearly evident fat. But you can't tell the calorie value of milk by the way it looks, Pat Bull reports. She often tests breast milk and finds it consistently higher in calories than formula (23).

The chart below compares the "draft" and "bottled" baby beverages.

A COMPARISON OF HUMAN MILK AND INFANT FORMULA

HUMAN MILK	INFANT FORMULA (cow milk and soy-based)
CALORIES	
The total number of calories from fat are about the same in human milk and cow milk. Typical human milk has about 21 calories per ounce.	Most formulas (prepared or reconstituted) have about 20 calories per ounce. Some special formulas have more (25–30 calories per ounce).
PROTEIN	
Human milk has a relatively low protein content, but the protein is well utilized. It is adequate to meet the protein needs of the baby until 6 months of age. From 6 to 11 months, most of the child's protein needs can be supplied from breast milk.	Cow milk contains about twice as much protein as human milk, but the protein is not absorbed as well as that of breast milk. Different ready-to-use formulas have protein of various types modified to be more absorbable.
Protein in human milk is easily digested. The sweet smell associated with breast-fed babies and the lack of odor in the stool, urine, and regurgitated milk indicates that the digestion and absorption of	Mixing formula concentrate according to directions is essential to provide the proper amount of protein.

HUMAN MILK	INFANT FORMULA (cow milk and soy-based)
the protein and fat are relatively complete (73).	
Breast milk contains proteins that protect infants against infection. Because human milk lacks beta-lactoglobulin, a common allergen, breast milk is the best protection against food allergies in infancy (184).	Formula contains no antiinfective proteins. Immunizing factors are less essential for the survival of babies born in the United States where the water supply is safe and there is far less exposure to polio, tuberculosis, and other diseases. Many bottle-fed babies are healthy without these immunizing factors.
The amino acids in human milk and cow milk are very different. Some suggest that human milk is better for premature or low-birth-weight babies. The milk of a woman who gives birth prematurely may be higher in protein than that of a woman who carries to term (131).	Infant formulas are now available that meet specific amino acid needs. Some formulas are designed to meet the needs of low-birth-weight babies.
Human milk contains large amounts of taurine, an amino acid needed for brain growth.	Cow milk has no taurine, although it is added to some formulas (108).

HUMAN MILK	INFANT FORMULA (cow milk and soy-based)
The type of fat in human milk is influenced by the mother's diet. If her diet is low in fat, the milk she produces will contain fat taken from the reserves of fat in her body.	Many formulas replace some of the saturated fat in cow milk with unsaturated and polyunsaturated vegetable oils such as soy oil.
Breast milk contains a substance that aids in rapid digestion and absorption of human milk fat (73). Human milk contains more cholesterol than cow milk.	Coconut oil, a saturated fat, is added to infant formulas to provide the medium and long-chain fatty acids in amounts comparable to those in human milk (106;178). Coconut oil containing fat blends and the fats in human milk are digested and absorbed similarly (61).
VITAMINS	
All the vitamins required for good nutrition and health care can be supplied in breast milk, with the possible exception of vitamin D if the baby is not routinely exposed to sunlight (108). The quantity of water-soluble vitamins is determined by the mother's intake of these vitamins.	Virtually all formulas are fortified with vitamin D. Vitamin K is routinely given to newborns to protect against hemorrhages. Most formulas are fortified with vitamins to ensure adequate nutrients for the baby.

HUMAN MILK	INFANT FORMULA (cow milk and soy-based)
MINERALS	
Mineral concentration is less in human milk than in cow milk, but this is easier on the newborn's kidneys.	Infant formulas are adjusted to lower the concentration of minerals in cow milk.
SODIUM	
Human milk contains less sodium than cow milk, reducing stress to an infant's kidneys. Maternal dietary sodium is unrelated to concentrations in milk (49).	Most formulas contain more sodium than found in human milk, but when manufacturers began removing salt from formula several years ago, some chloride deficiencies developed, so it was restored. The level appears to be suitable now.
FLUORIDE	
During the first months, when babies are fed exclusively with breast milk, they generally are not given water (23). The American Academy of Pediatrics recommends supplements for breast-fed babies living in areas where water is not fluoridated (171).	Concentrated formulas contain very low levels of fluoride to prevent overdoses in areas where formula is prepared with fluoridated water. If formula is made with unfluoridated water, or a ready-to-use formula is used, a supplement may be given.

HUMAN MILK	INFANT FORMULA (cow milk and soy-based)
ZINC	
There is a high concentration of zinc in colostrum; in later milk the levels are lower, but absorption rate is high (41%) (125).	The level is similar to human milk, but the absorption rate is lower (31% from standard formulas, 14% from soy formulas).
IRON	
The infant exclusively breast-fed for the first 6 months is not at risk of iron deficiency anemia or depletion of iron stores (45). Babies who are being breast-fed should not be given supplementary foods during the first four months of life. After that time, they will need iron from fortified cereals and other iron-fortified foods.	The iron level in regular cow milk is low. The American Academy of Pediatrics recommends that iron-fortified formula be used for all formula-fed infants. Fortification protects against anemia (38). There is no evidence that the iron in infant formulas causes stomachaches or intestinal problems (158).
When exclusively breast-fed, infants absorb the iron in breast milk very efficiently. Absorption is promoted by vitamin C and lactose in breast milk (108).	Babies generally drink an amount of formula that will provide adequate iron (158).

HUMAN MILK	INFANT FORMULA (cow milk and soy-based)
CALCIUM	
The baby receives calcium in breast milk even when the mother does not consume adequate calcium, but in that case some is drawn from her bones (108).	The high level of calcium in cow milk is reduced in infant formulas to levels well accepted by babies.

In 1980, the Food and Drug Administration passed a law to ensure that every precaution be taken to make infant formula safe. The number of healthy children in this country who have been bottle-fed is a testimony to the safety and effectiveness of infant formulas.

The human milk of well-nourished mothers is used as the standard to determine the adequacy of infant formulas. Modern technology has made great strides in formulating human-milk substitutes. We do not, however, know the long-term effects of substances that are added to formulas, such as emulsifiers, thickening agents, antioxidants, and pH adjusters; no ill effects are currently recognized. Moreover, there may be some properties in human milk that have not yet been discovered.

HOLDING THE BABY DURING FEEDINGS

Parents of both breast- and bottle-fed babies should make a special point of holding and cuddling their babies during the important first weeks. Babies do not thrive on milk alone!

Mothers and fathers usually experience an intense feeling of attachment—the term *bonding* has been used to define the phenomenon—when the baby is breast-fed, but it is not exclusive to breast-feeding. Bonding is the result of physical contact—holding, touching, smelling, stroking, rocking, feeding. It is best skin-on-skin, with the baby cuddled against parent or parents and encircled in their arms.

Bonding has long-term effects. A study conducted over a period of five years compared mothers and infants who had an additional sixteen hours or more of close contact during the first three days after birth with a group that did not have the extra contact. After two years, mothers in the extra-contact group seemed more interested in their children's development. They used more complex language in talking with their children and spent time explaining cause and effect (134). Certainly bonding is reinforced during the holding and cuddling of a bottle-fed baby. While many people think of bonding as a maternal phenomenon, fathers and other family members also bond by holding and cuddling newborn children.

Many hospitals now have "rooming in," or some provision for mother and father (and sometimes other family members) to hold and care for the baby soon after birth. This arrangement promotes bonding. Talk to your doctor about this early in your pregnancy. You may want to plan delivery at a hospital where your baby can stay with you rather than in a separate nursery. This arrangement may not be possible if either mother or baby needs special medical attention, but you may not know this until after delivery.

THE MOTHER'S EXPERIENCE OF BREAST-FEEDING

Mothers find that nursing helps maintain the sense of attachment that develops during pregnancy. "Breast-feeding was a very special experience because it was something only I could do for my baby," one mother told us. "I felt good because I was giving her the very best start."

Yes, breast-feeding does take time, energy, and commitment. It ties a mother down, especially during the first month or so until the process is established. Some women enjoy breast-feeding for just these reasons. It's a "nesting" time and mothers want to focus attention on the new baby.

The most enthusiastic proponents of breast-feeding are women who have successfully nursed their children. Some may be almost *too* enthusiastic! The reason is that for many, it is an extremely emotional—and physically exciting—experience.

For Anne, it was very strange—and not always wonderful: "No one told me that I would be in pain *after* the baby was born: The episiotomy hurt, my breasts were hot and tender, my nipples were sensitive, and I got very little sleep. But the feeling of the milk let-down—that tingling sensation—is one I'll never forget. The reality of the baby close to me as I nursed her overwhelmed me. I knew I wanted her and I wanted to nurture her. I was doing something no one else could do."

For many women, modesty is a consideration in the decision whether to feed her child at the breast. But no one says you have to make a production of nursing your baby in public. Most women prefer to nurse privately.

If you can't find a private spot, you can nurse discreetly by adjusting your clothing or covering your breast with a blanket or cloth diaper. Much of the self-consciousness women experience when they first begin nursing is lost as they become more comfortable with it and it begins to feel more natural. Few situations occur in which you and baby cannot find a quiet, private place to nurse.

Some men are uncomfortable witnessing breast-feeding because they see their partner's breasts only within a sexual context. The idea of fondling a milk-filled breast may seem repulsive, or it may be a real turn-on.

There is an unmistakable connection between breast-feeding and sex. Nursing is sexually arousing because both activities stimulate the same hormones and involve the same nerves. Milk may drip from the breasts during lovemaking. When nursing, the uterus contracts, a natural phenomenon that helps return it to normal size. These contractions may feel very sensual.

Some new mothers become preoccupied with nursing and lose interest in sex. (This can be helpful because sexual intercourse is usually not recommended for a few weeks after childbirth.) Actually, the changes and adjustments a woman makes when she gives birth may temporarily turn off desire, regardless of the way she feeds her baby. These are the times to show love by hugging, kissing, back rubbing, and stroking the baby together.

Another concern women have about breast-feeding is the effect it may have on the breasts. While nursing does change the breasts temporarily, if you wear a well-fitted bra, your breasts will not sag and they will return to their prepregnancy size and shape when the baby is about nine months old. Many women's breasts permanently increase in size as a result of pregnancy, even if they choose not to breast-feed.

The size and shape of a woman's breasts make little difference to her success in nursing. Nature has determined that every mother, with few exceptions, can nurse her offspring. A woman who has inverted nipples, or who suspects that she has any barrier to breast-feeding, should consult her doctor early in pregnancy about techniques that will prepare her for nursing.

If you do not breast-feed, your breasts will fill with milk and become engorged for several days after delivery. Lactation-suppressing drugs may be given but the trend today is to do without them (170). Women who choose not to breast-feed are advised to wear a well-fitting bra and, if there is pain, use ice packs and take a pain reliever such as acetaminophen. The pain is rarely severe enough to require stronger treatment (170).

DOING WHAT DOESN'T COME NATURALLY

Breast-feeding is a *learned* skill; it does not come naturally. Dr. Dana Raphael, an anthropologist, noted that in cultures where women breast-feed their babies, a system of training and support exists. A helper assists the new mother and teaches her the art of mothering (148). The helper may pitch in with the household chores, but her primary task is to teach the new mother the tricks of caring for and feeding her baby.

In our society, your helper may be a friend or relative who can provide practical tips on breast-feeding and child care and give encouragement during the first weeks. The La Leche League is the best-known support group. They offer information and support through local groups and publish many books and pamphlets. Local hospitals and women's health centers now have support groups. Certified lactation consultants, identified by the initials I.B.C.L.C. (International Board of Certified Lactation Consultants), offer information and individualized instruction. Sometimes a registered dietitian can provide advice and counsel. Your local hospital can give you names and addresses.

If you decide to breast-feed, you will want a physician who is supportive during your pregnancy. Unfortunately, many health practitioners have not had specific training related to lactation. You might ask, when you are in the process of choosing a doctor, how many of his or her patients breast-feed, whether breast-feeding preparation is included in the doctor's prenatal care, and whether you will have an opportunity to nurse your baby immediately after delivery and on demand during your hospital stay. Because babies nurse better if their mothers have not been heavily sedated during delivery, you should ask your doctor about the type of anesthetic to be used during delivery. While your doctor may give you medication for pain, drugs that interfere with the initiation of breast-feeding can generally be avoided.

Women who require cesarean deliveries can successfully breast-feed soon after the baby is born. It helps ease the disappointment that some women feel when they are unable to deliver vaginally as planned, especially if they have prepared for a natural childbirth delivery. Discuss this possibility so you will know the degree to which the doctor will cooperate with your commitment to breast-feed.

TIME TO FEED

New babies require a great deal of time and attention. The amount of milk newborns consume at first is limited by the size of their stomachs to only one to three ounces. Newborn babies frequently nurse every hour and a half to three hours for periods of five to ten minutes or longer. Bottle-fed babies typically want to be fed every three to four hours. Infant formula produces a curd in the infant's stomach that is larger than that produced by breast milk. The larger curd satisfies the baby longer than the smaller curd (23). Many infants are gassy or coliky because of their immature digestive systems. Sometimes a doctor will change formulas if one is not easily handled by the baby.

Think of feeding times as rest time for Mom. Put your feet up and relax during feeding. Talk and sing to your baby. Enjoy the thrill of having your baby gaze at your face and of capturing one another's eye. Let your mate, mother, or a high-school helper vacuum, wash, and get dinner ready if you are feeding your baby. If your mate, a family member, or friend is bottle-feeding your baby, take the time to rest anyway.

You may find it frightening to contemplate caring for a baby if you already have another child, especially if that child is a preschooler. You've no doubt heard it said that the first baby takes all of your time, and somehow the babies who follow just fit in. The first baby is the most time-consuming because you are learning; subsequent children are generally easier. Twins take all of your time, and you may need help—especially to fit in needed rest!

If you breast-feed, the preparation of food takes no time at all, and you can leave off and resume, if necessary, to meet the immediate needs of other children. The milk will be fresh and ready whenever you and your baby get together. But you must be there and ready to feed. For day and night feedings alike, both the responsibility and the joy of nourishing will be yours. Other family members can hold and care for the baby at other times.

One father told us, "All this talk of fathers of breast-fed babies not having to get up in the night is nonsense! When the baby cried, I'd get up and change her, then bring her into our bed to be nursed. I remember thinking my wife had the easy part; she never had to get up!"

If you bottle-feed, you will have to spend some time preparing the bottles. Although prepared infant formula is sterile in the can, most pediatricians recommend sterilizing equipment during the early weeks. You will have to boil water or use special bottled "baby water" to mix with concentrated or powdered formula. All formula must be carefully prepared according to directions. A hungry baby doesn't want to wait for you to stir and mix and pour and heat! In spite of what others do, you should not heat bottles in a microwave oven. Many babies have suffered serious burns from formula heated in a microwave (88). That's because the formula is unevenly heated and can be very hot, even when the bottle is only warm to the touch. So add a couple of minutes to preparation time to heat the bottle in an electric warmer, in water on the stove, or under hot running water. If you don't want to bother, see if your baby will be happy with milk straight out of the fridge. Babies can get used to milk warm or chilled!

When Mary's daughter Rachel was born, Mary decided to bottle-feed, a choice supported by her husband, her mother, and the woman who took care of the baby during the day if Mary was working and didn't take Rachel along. "Peter and I worked out a system with both of our children. I fed the baby a bottle late at night before I went to sleep. Then Peter would feed the baby if she woke during the night and again before he left for work, while I was still sleeping."

Peter says, "I had a special time with my daughters and developed a wonderful closeness with them during those nighttime hours in the easy chair. It wasn't long before the night feedings stopped, but the nighttime routine remained. Throughout the early years, if Rachel or Leslie woke, they stood in their cribs and called 'Daddy.' "

BACK TO WORK

Three generations ago, a woman who worked outside the home violated the norm. But today economic necessity and a new ethic that supports and encourages women to work in order to fulfill their intellectual, emotional, and economic potential mean that most women hold jobs outside the home. In some circles, women who have decided to stay at home and raise children have been made to feel inadequate. Many professional women opt to take off some time to be with infants; others choose to return to work for economic or other reasons.

While bias against employed mothers may still exist among some pediatricians, professional organizations acknowledge the trend. The Committee on Psychosocial Aspects of Child and Family Health of the Academy of Pediatrics urges pediatricians to support subsidized parental leaves, encourage active participation of fathers in child and household care, and assist in helping parents to find high-quality substitute care (2). The American College of Obstetrics and Gynecology encourages physicians to help prepare patients who plan an early return to work (4).

If you plan to return to work, find a physician who will help you to provide a smooth transition. You'll have greater peace of mind if you have a doctor who will be available to those who care for your child in your absence. Women who plan to breast-feed after returning to work or school should also find a physician who will be supportive. In practical terms, this means counseling regarding pumping and storing milk and avoiding exhaustion. If you plan to wean your baby before going back to work, you'll need information and support from both your doctor and the baby's doctor. Some women get a lot of help from lactation counselors or breast-feeding support groups.

The business community is gradually changing its attitudes about parenting. Some companies now give paternity leave when a baby is born; others have extended maternity benefits. More mothers are returning to work on a part-time or job-sharing basis. Many jobs that use computers allow women to work full-time at a home computer and use technology to connect the offices. On-site day-care facilities encourage women to return to work full-time. Thus, breast-feeding and working away from home are more doable than ever before. But it still isn't easy.

When you first announce your pregnancy, your employer may ask about your plans to return to work. Before you commit yourself, evaluate your company's policies and programs for working mothers. It's up to you, not your employer, to figure out how you can be both a competent worker and mother. How you handle feeding will be part of the plan you formulate.

- Evaluate your current job responsibilities. Some situations require your presence full time; others allow more flexibility. Is travel a part of your job? Do you have regular work hours? Can you do work at home? Will your schedule allow you time for nursing or pumping? Can you combine breast- and bottle-feeding?

- What kind of child care will you use? If you have regular working hours, work and baby schedules go smoothly. But if you have a job in which overtime is likely or you need flexible working hours, you may need to consider live-in help or willing and flexible relatives or friends to keep peace on both fronts.

  It is easier to continue breast-feeding if your company provides on-site day care and your schedule allows for it. If your child is near enough for you to go back and forth to work quickly, you can breast-feed before and after work, and supplement with either expressed milk or formula when you are away.
- Is there a place at work where you can express breast milk, if you decide to do so? During the first three months, you will need to pump your milk twice a day if you are away from your baby; from three to five months you will have to do it once a day. After that time, your milk supply will be adequate to nurse morning and night without pumping (23).

  Some companies now have electric pumping machines in a lounge especially for lactating women. The Y-pump is quick and easy to use. In twenty minutes or less, while she eats her lunch, takes a break, or catches up on required reading (the pump leaves both hands free), a woman can extract about eight ounces of milk. The double pump that stimulates both breasts simultaneously produces more milk in a shorter period of time than other pumping methods (108).

  Smaller electric pumps are available for rent. You will need a place that is comfortable and private, where you can relax so your milk will flow freely. A private office is ideal. If you don't have an office of your own, ask the personnel director if there is an empty office available, preferably one with a door that can be locked for privacy. Some employers have a health service or athletic facilities with suitable space. Hand-expressing milk in a public restroom or toilet stall is less conducive to success.

You will also need a place to chill the expressed milk. A refrigerator is best, but if one isn't available, you can use an insulated container.

- Develop and present a plan to your employer. One of the biggest problems associated with maternity leave is that women do not stick to the terms of the agreement. Many women find that it's harder to return to work than they anticipated it would be. They delay their return, want part-time work when they committed to full-time, or decide not to return at all. This behavior isn't fair to employers who have kept a position open, asked others to cover for you during your leave, or hired temporary help in your absence.

One mother we know was determined to nurse her baby after she returned to her job as a fashion reporter on the staff of a local newspaper. She had a flexible schedule, allowing for occasional late arrivals and early departures, as well as time midday to express milk for the next day. She had an office where this could be done discreetly. She also had a small refrigerator in her office where she could store the milk. She nursed her daughter for a year. Nursing was her way of feeling close to her baby.

It's easy to conclude that decreased breast-feeding in this country is caused by increased maternal employment, but studies show that, overall, breast-feeding and employment are not mutually exclusive, though women who work tend to wean sooner. In 1987, the Ross Laboratories Mothers' Survey, mailed quarterly to 155,000 mothers of six-month-old babies, reported that initially the same percentage (55 percent) of both working and nonworking women chose to breast-feed their newborns. But six months later, only 10 percent of full-time working mothers were still breast-feeding (154).

Women do not necessarily stop breast-feeding when they return to work. Those who nurse for at least four to six weeks and have firmly established lactation tend to be highly motivated to continue after returning to work (202). They often show great determination in working out the complexities of scheduling and child care, finding ways to pump milk, and dealing with the stress that comes from trying to manage both work and home (108).

Women *do* continue to carry 70 percent to 80 percent of the child care and household duties when both parents work (108). This is the subject of much discussion and negotiation in many families.

If you take pride in being in control over what you do and when you do it, a baby may really throw you. Breast-feeding puts additional responsibility on a mother and demands time and planning. For many, infant formula is a better choice because it promotes peace of mind with less need to alter workdays and express and store milk. Bottle-feeding allows others to feed your baby and relieves you of the sole responsibility, while still meeting the baby's nutritional and developmental needs.

WORKDAY BREAST-FEEDING SCHEDULE

Morning	Allow 45 minutes to an hour for a relaxed feeding. You may want to bathe or shower and lay out your clothes for work the night before. Let your mate fix breakfast and care for other children. If care is not at your home, bring the baby to the day-care provider. Allow time to give your sitter (or the day-care center staff) an update on particular concerns (how the baby slept and ate, bowel movements, reactions to shots, etc.). Leave expressed milk for feeding your baby. Be sure it is kept chilled to stay fresh.
Through the day	For the first three months, you will have to pump your milk twice a day—say at 11:00 A.M. and 2:00 P.M. After that, one midday pumping will be adequate.

Returning home	Tell the sitter to delay feeding until you get there, if at all possible. Then nurse your baby at the sitter's or as soon as you get home.
Evenings/Nights	Babies of working mothers sleep more during the day but want to be fed at night. The extra feeding stimulates and maintains the mother's supply of milk.
Days Off	You may want to provide extra feedings, but many mothers continue the weekday routine to allow themselves time for rest and relaxation. If possible, someone other than mother should give the bottles. Mother smells like milk!

MAKING THE TRANSITION FROM BREAST TO BOTTLE

Many women want to breast-feed, but don't like the idea of being tied down continually. There are still a few die-hard breast-feeding advocates who would never let their baby's lips touch a bottle. And it is true that babies who are given bottles before being well established at the breast sometimes become confused when presented the alternative. This happens because two very different sucking techniques are used for breast and bottle, and the very young baby may not master both simultaneously.

The time to introduce a nursing baby to a bottle is when the baby is about four weeks old. Then you can give one or two bottles a week without interfering with nursing. Most babies are flexible and will adjust to an occasional bottle of either expressed breast milk or infant formula. And knowing that a bottle can be given may provide you with peace of mind.

During the first six weeks, babies who receive formula regularly but who are still nursed may begin to show a definite preference for the bottle. Formula flows much more quickly and with less effort from the bottle. Some eager eaters like this (23).

It isn't just babies but nursing mothers who may experience confusion if bottles are given too early or too often. The bottle is more likely to interfere if the mother is not confident about having enough milk. Babies fed infant formula that has a larger curd than breast milk tend to go longer between feedings—a tempting advantage for a weary parent. Some women find they enjoy having others share in the feeding process. Fathers and grandparents usually love sharing the role!

You may choose to breast-feed for only a few weeks or months. To breast-feed, even for a short time, is good for the baby. If you switch from breast to bottle at any time during the first year, your baby should be given an appropriate infant formula chosen by your doctor.

If you give a breast-fed baby solid foods before four months of age, you will be replacing what is nutritionally ideal with nutritionally imperfect food for that stage of baby's development. Moreover, babies who are given solids too early are more likely to develop food allergies (158). Although many people believe it, there is no evidence that early introduction of solid food will pacify a fussy baby or will make a baby sleep better.

BREAST-FEEDING AND YOUR DIET

Nature has a will for babies to survive. A mother can produce adequate milk for her baby, whether she is thin, obese, short, small-breasted, or even poorly nourished. The major determinant of milk production is how much the baby demands (171). A big, hungry baby may want as much as thirty-four or thirty-six ounces a day; a smaller baby wants less. If you nurse twins, you'll be able to make more milk than if you nurse a single baby.

Stress, fatigue, illness, dieting, and excessive alcohol consumption can influence milk production, but inadequate sucking is the main reason for an insufficient supply of milk. Sucking stimulates the mammary glands. If you have to be away from your baby for long periods of time during the first few months after giving birth, it's hard to maintain an adequate supply unless you regularly pump your milk. Pumping, like sucking, stimulates milk production.

In spite of what you may have heard, drinking beer does not aid nursing, and neither does drinking water. Fluids consumed in excess of thirst will not increase the amount of milk you can produce (173). Alcohol isn't recommended for lactating women, but it seems that small amounts will not harm a baby. The amount is determined by body size. A 132-pound woman, for instance, can occasionally have up to two and one-half ounces of liquor, eight ounces of wine, or two cans of beer. Excessive alcohol consumption reduces the volume and interferes with milk release (173). Regular alcohol consumption of more than one drink a day may damage the baby's development as alcohol is transfered into breast milk.

In a major 1991 report on nutrition during lactation, a committee of experts found that even though a mother's diet may be less than what's recommended, human milk consistently supplies carbohydrate, fat, protein, and most minerals to meet an infant's needs. The vitamin composition of the milk, however, is more directly related to what the mother eats (173).

Most advice about breast-feeding focuses on what's good for the baby. But how does nursing affect the mother's nutrition and health? Consider what it takes for an exclusively breast-fed baby to double its weight in the first four to six months after birth! The mother's whole body is influenced by lactation. Without adequate "nutritional fuel," breast-feeding diverts nutrients away from the mother's physiologic needs, depletes her nutrient reserves, and robs her body tissues. A mother's diet may not greatly influence the composition of breast milk, but it surely affects a breast-feeding woman's health and well-being. Pregnancies close together can magnify the stress on her body.

Women who are anxious to get back to their prepregnancy size will need a well-defined eating plan to meet their own goals for weight loss without compromising their own and their baby's nutritional status.

Calories

Some of the extra pounds gained during pregnancy are insurance that calories will be present for production of breast milk. But the energy needed for lactation comes from additional calories from food, not the mobilization of leftover body fat from pregnancy. Breast-feeding is not a quick weight-loss plan. On average, new mothers lose one to two pounds a month after the first month, whether or not they breast-feed. As many as 20 percent of nursing mothers maintain or gain weight (173).

It takes 400 to 700 calories a day to make an adequate supply of milk (158). The RDAs recommend an increase of 500 calories (above the nonpregnant need) in the mother's diet. For women who were underweight or whose weight gain during pregnancy was low, an increase of 650 calories a day is recommended during the first six months of breast-feeding. Lactating women who get enough calories are likely to obtain all nutrients, with the exception of calcium and zinc (173). Women who have a high level of physical activity also need more calories.

A breast-feeding mother who eats less than fifteen hundred calories a day will find herself fatigued and may be unable to produce enough milk to nourish her baby. A weight loss of more than four and a half pounds a month can inhibit milk production (173). Strict dieting is not recommended for *any* new mother, even if she is bottle-feeding. The first six to eight weeks is an emotionally fragile time, and dieting may bring on depression and add physiologic stress to an already stressful time.

IMPLICATIONS FOR FOOD CHOICES

Continue to eat a variety of nutritious foods but find sources of sugar and fat that can be eliminated. Identify low-fat products that contain the key nutrients most likely to be in short supply, like lean meat (iron and zinc) and skim milk (calcium). If breast-feeding is well established and the baby is growing well after six weeks, breast-feeding mothers can cut one hundred calories a day from their intake.

Protein

Most human milk contains enough protein to meet the needs of the baby's growth until about six months old. Protein is generally not a concern because most women in this country consume more than enough protein.

There is no specific place in the body to store protein for emergency use. So when protein is withdrawn from stores, it means that your muscles and vital organs lose part of their structural protein.

IMPLICATIONS FOR FOOD CHOICES

While women need slightly more protein during lactation than during pregnancy, the amount is easily attainable especially if you continue to drink milk. For the first six months of lactation sixty-five grams per day is advised, sixty-two grams per day in the second six months of lactation.

Fat

There are no recommendations for fat intake during lactation, but the amount of saturated or polyunsaturated fat the nursing mother consumes is reflected in the fat composition in her milk. Polyunsaturated dietary fat is a source of essential fatty acids, which pass through to the baby.

Cholesterol

The cholesterol content of milk is not affected by a mother's diet. The amount of cholesterol in breast milk drops as lactation progresses, even though fat increases (202). Early in lactation, the cholesterol helps the baby's brain cells to develop.

IMPLICATIONS FOR FOOD CHOICES

Cutting total fat is a good way to cut calories and cholesterol without jeopardizing nutritional needs during lactation.

Vitamins

The breast-fed baby depends on the mother's diet to provide water-soluble vitamins, especially vitamins C, B_6, thiamin, and riboflavin. The human lactation system processes the fragile water-soluble vitamins in your diet so that maximum amounts are passed to the nursing baby.

The vitamin A in mother's milk is strongly influenced by her diet (202). Both a woman's intake of dietary vitamin D and her exposure to ultraviolet sunlight influence the vitamin D in breast milk. While there is no total agreement, most doctors prescribe vitamin D to breast-fed babies to promote the growth of strong bones (74). Human milk contains more vitamin E than cow milk does, and virtually all formulas contain added vitamin E. Virtually all American babies, whether breast- or bottle-fed, get an injection of vitamin K at birth to avoid blood-clotting problems until the baby's digestive tract begins to make vitamin K (182).

Folate levels in red blood cells of women who breast-feed for more than six months can be as much as 30 percent less than normal, indicating the extent to which this vitamin's reserves have been depleted.

IMPLICATIONS FOR FOOD CHOICES

Most vitamins are needed in larger amounts during lactation than during pregnancy. The nutrient with the biggest increase is vitamin C; this need can be easily met with the selection of two good vitamin C sources a day from the list in chapter 5. Continue to drink milk fortified with vitamin D. Nursing mothers should try to get their vitamins from foods rather than supplements.

Minerals

IRON

The amount of iron is breast milk is low and is not affected by the mother's diet. This is generally not of great concern because full-term babies are born with iron stores to last several months. The mother's need for iron during the postpartum period, however, is a matter of concern. Because so many women have depleted iron reserves after giving birth, iron supplements are generally prescribed or prenatal supplements continued for three to four months after birth. A blood test two days after delivery may indicate whether supplements are recommended. Women recover some iron as the expanded blood volume of pregnancy returns to normal, and while there is some bleeding after delivery, women don't lose iron through menstruation for the first months (or longer if they breast-feed) after giving birth.

FLUORIDE

Fluoride concentrations in breast milk are related to the mother's intake of fluoride unless the amount is very high (1.4 parts per million) (173). The American Academy of Pediatrics recommends fluoride supplements for breast-fed babies if they do not drink fluoridated water or formula prepared with fluoridated water.

CALCIUM

The calcium level of human milk is relatively constant regardless of the mother's diet (56). But the mother who doesn't get enough dietary calcium risks having the calcium in her bones raided to maintain the levels in her milk, thus weakening her bone strength and making her more susceptible to osteoporosis later in life. Calcium is a greater concern for younger women who breast-feed, since the calcium content of bones increases until age twenty-five. During lactation, continue to include the lowfat milk and yogurt, or other calcium-rich foods in your diet you've learned to love during pregnancy unless you have a medical reason to stop drinking milk.

Liquids

In spite of what you may have heard, a woman does not need to drink inordinate amounts of liquid when she is breast-feeding. No evidence exists that drinking more water or any other fluid will increase the amount of milk produced (56). When any fluid leaves the body, however, it draws on the bloodstream and body cells to release water. Thus, the production of milk creates a need for fluid. Thirst is the body's signal to replace liquid. Milk and fruit juices provide not only water but extra vitamins and minerals needed during breast-feeding. Large amounts of caffeine-containing beverages may keep both you and baby awake. In spite of what you may have heard, beer does not increase milk production, and it no longer contains brewer's yeast, a source of B vitamins. Beer does provide fluid and its alcohol content causes some women to relax, but it is *not* a nutritious beverage.

A study of four hundred breast-fed infants published in the *New England Journal of Medicine* (1989) showed that when mothers had more than one drink a day, it had a slight but significant detrimental effect on the child's motor development, but not mental development, at age one year (113). There is no evidence that an occasional drink has any negative effect. After a nursing woman drinks liquor, her breast milk contains levels of ethanol similar to those in her blood. Curiously, acetaldehyde, a highly toxic substance in liquor, does not appear in mother's milk (202).

Vegetarian Nursing Mothers

A sensible vegetarian diet that includes sufficient calories and protein is adequate for both mother and baby during lactation. The mother needs to pay special attention to her intake of calcium and iron. If she eats no animal products, she may need a B_{12} supplement to prevent anemia in both herself and her baby. If she does not drink milk, the calcium sources she used during pregnancy should be continued.

Vegetarian mothers should be encouraged to consume their extra calories from foods that are sources of high-quality protein such as grains, nuts, vegetables, legumes, and dairy products.

If a breast-feeding vegetarian mother wants to supplement with formula that doesn't contain cow milk, she may want to ask her doctor if soy-based formula is appropriate for her baby.

Dietary Supplements for Breast-Feeding Women

Many lactating women are advised to continue taking prenatal supplements during the first few months of breastfeeding. But most experts contend that increased needs can be met by a well-balanced diet. The only exception, for most women, is in iron intake. Supplemental iron to replenish stores lost in pregnancy is wise for all postpartum women, whether they breast- or bottle-feed their infants. Otherwise, eating a balanced diet is the best way to stay healthy.

CONTAMINANTS IN BREAST MILK

Breast milk is not always 100 percent pure. The composition of the milk reflects the environment and the mother's personal habits, which in some cases may not be the best habits for growing babies. We discussed the effects of caffeine and alcohol in chapter 7. The conscientious mother wants to know about any substance that is potentially harmful to her baby. Possible exposure to any of these substances may influence your decision about how to feed your child.

Caffeine or Coffee

Caffeine is transmitted through breast milk. Infants exposed to high levels or frequent doses may be irritable or wakeful, but the caffeine in one or two cups of coffee won't affect a nursing baby. Large intakes of coffee, even decaffeinated coffee, may reduce the iron content of breast milk (173).

Nicotine

In humans and in experiments with animals, heavy smoking reduces the amount of milk produced (133). There are reports that three- and four-day-old babies of breast-feeding mothers who smoked from six to sixteen cigarettes a day refused to suck, became apathetic, vomited, and retained urine and stools. Breast-fed babies of women who smoke breathe more smoke than they consume in breast milk (54). While bottle-fed babies are not influenced by nicotine in milk, they do not breathe in smoke. Mothers and caregivers should not smoke when holding an infant.

Marijuana and Cocaine

The most active ingredient in marijuana is fat-soluble and therefore passes along in breast milk. Babies born to women who use cocaine generally have multiple complications that may make it impossible for them to be breast-fed. Cases have been reported in which babies have reacted to cocaine in their mother's milk by showing symptoms of cocaine intoxication (28). One baby developed seizures when cocaine was used as a topical anesthetic for nipple soreness (27).

Drugs

Before you take *any* drug, prescription or over-the-counter, be sure to find out if it is passed through breast milk and poses a threat to the nursing infant. The infant's kidneys and liver may be unable to excrete or detoxify these drugs. If you choose to breast-feed, ask your doctor or pharmacist for a list of permitted over-the-counter drugs and take no prescription drugs without specific advice that they are safe for your baby. The best guide is *Drugs in Pregnancy and Lactation* (18), a comprehensive manual that is used by physicians and pharmacists.

Many common drugs such as aspirin, Valium, and a variety of antibiotics can be dangerous if you are breast-feeding. Even taking large amounts of aspirin, which is usually safe, can cause your newborn baby to hemorrhage (177).

Some women have been advised to wean if they require medications, but this does not take into account the mother's feelings about weaning, the baby's experience if suddenly taken from the breast, or the loss to the baby of the beneficial ingredients in mother's milk. Ask your physician if there is another way to treat the illness, or if simply waiting it out with no medication is a real threat to your health. Sometimes breast milk is pumped and discarded and formula is given as a temporary measure. Then breast-feeding is resumed after the medication is stopped.

Many drugs have little or no effect on the nursing infant because they do not pass into milk. With some drugs, however, the effects may appear to be minimal yet trace amounts absorbed by the baby can lead to an allergic reaction to that drug at a later time (82).

If you must take medicine, take it just after nursing so levels will be reduced before the next session.

Environmental Contaminants

There has been a great deal of concern about environmental contaminants in breast milk. The public has been alarmed to learn of incidences of cancer and birth defects where high levels of contaminants are found in the breast milk of women.

With the awareness of the health hazard posed by contaminants, their use in North America has diminished greatly in recent years. In our search of the literature, we were unable to find documentation of dangerously high levels of PCBs (polychlorinated biphenyls) or DDT in the diets of American women except among women who regularly worked with these compounds or ate fish caught in contaminated waters.

Levels of insecticides in human milk vary with the weight of the mother and the duration of nursing. Levels are higher at the end of a feeding when the fat content of the milk is high (173). Insecticide levels are generally minimal and not a concern.

Heavy metals, such as lead, mercury, and arsenic, are greater in certain water supplies, cow milk, and formula reconstituted with tap water than in human milk (173).

If there is a question about breast milk contamination, ask your state health department for help. Risks posed by contaminated well water or fishing water tend to be confined to local areas. Doctors generally agree that the benefits of breast-feeding greatly outweigh the risks of environmental contaminants except for individual women exposed to high levels of a specific contaminant.

There are several things you can do to minimize the potential of adding contaminants to your diet.

- Wash fruits and vegetables thoroughly.
- Since PCBs are found in fat, decrease fat in your diet.
- Avoid crash diets, which release large amounts of stored fats and hence possible stored toxicants from previous exposures.

- Do not eat fish or shellfish from lakes and rivers that have been contaminated by PCBs or other chemicals
- Avoid exposure to industrial chemicals, pesticides, and "carbon" paper that contains no carbons (184).

OTHER SUBSTANCES TO AVOID WHILE BREAST-FEEDING

Oral Contraceptives

A number of studies have shown that traditional oral contraceptives containing both estrogen and progestin reduce the quantity and quality of breast milk. Talk to your doctor about desirable methods of contraception while you are still nursing your baby.

Food Additives and Artificial Sweeteners

Very little is known about specific food additives or artificial sweeteners and their potential for transmittal through breast milk. Relying primarily on less processed foods without large amounts of additives is wise whether breast-feeding or not. A varied diet reduces the amount of any one food eaten and protects you and your baby from large quantities of additives.

Foods that Cause Gas

If your baby has gas, don't blame it on something *you* ate! During the first months, a baby's digestive system is very immature, and gas forms easily. Large amounts of lactose, most notably found in milk, may irritate some babies. If a baby is fussy after the mother eats strongly flavored food, it's probably because he or she does not like the *flavor* the food gives to breast milk.

THE BOTTLE-FED BABY

All infant formulas are not the same. If you decide to bottle-feed while you are in the hospital, the doctor (usually the pediatrician) will order a specific formula based on your baby's weight, family history of allergies, and other factors. The baby will be observed to be sure that the formula is well tolerated. The real test will be whether your child does well on it during his or her first weeks and months. If there are problems, another formula will be substituted.

Most liquid formulas contain about twenty calories per ounce. Some formulas with more calories per ounce are used for low-birth-weight babies and babies who have sucking or eating problems. Formulas differ in sources of protein, fat, and carbohydrate. Doctors usually prescribe formulas fortified with iron.

Most popular commercial formulas come in a concentrate to which boiled tap or bottled water is added, or in ready-to-serve form that you pour directly into a clean bottle. Bottles can be prepared singly or for a whole day. They must be refrigerated once they are prepared. Ready-to-serve formula also comes in expensive but handy disposable bottles that do not require refrigeration. If you are traveling with a bottle-fed baby, bring along ready-to-serve formula of the type usually used.

It is not necessary to warm formulas as long as the baby is

happy with its temperature. Babies used to room-temperature formula like it that way; babies used to chilled formulas like it that way. If it makes *you* feel better to give your baby a warm bottle, then do so. You can warm it up by running it under hot water for a minute or two, by warming in a pan of water on the stove, or by using an electric bottle-warmer. As mentioned earlier, do not warm bottles in the microwave. The milk will not be evenly heated and may scald your baby's mouth. However you heat a bottle of formula, shake it well and test the temperature on the back of your hand. Curiously, the traditional wrist-test uses a part of your body that is less sensitive to heat.

The most important aspect of formula preparation is sanitation. The bottles and nipples must be absolutely clean; the top of a liquid formula should be wiped clean before opening. Virtually all women who give infant formulas in the United States use a commercially prepared formula. Because it is sterile in the can, you only need to add clean water to clean bottles. Using ready-to-serve formula assures cleanliness of the product until it leaves the can. Also, appropriate amounts of vitamins and minerals have already been added. Mixing and sterilizing mixtures of evaporated milk, sweetener, and water is a thing of the past.

Always read formula directions carefully. If you use concentrated formula, add the *correct* amount of bottled or clean water. Formula that is too concentrated or too weak can cause your baby serious problems. If you have someone else feed your baby, prepare the bottles yourself or watch the preparer to make sure it's done properly. If you are using ready-to-serve formula or disposable bottles there is less chance of error. The formula in an opened can may be kept, refrigerated, for no more than twenty-four hours. Milk left from one feeding should not be saved for another feeding, no matter how wasteful that may seem. Bacteria from the baby's mouth contaminates the formula and can cause illness if it is saved and offered at the next meal.

Two rules that come automatically with breast-feeding also can be practiced when you bottle-feed your baby.

1. Do not overfeed. Do not try to make your baby empty the bottle. This practice fosters eating past satisfaction and increases the possibility of weight-control problems throughout life. Breast-fed babies decide when to stop sucking, and that's that.

Newborns typically take twenty to thirty minutes to finish a bottle. If a newborn finishes a bottle in under fifteen minutes, a nipple with a smaller hole may be necessary.

Newborns may consume as little as one ounce or as much as four ounces. Larger, active babies generally take more formula than smaller babies, and fussy babies want to be fed more often. If your baby refuses to take any more formula, he or she may be full. Let your baby be the judge. If this happens consistently, pour less formula into bottles.

2. Hold and cuddle the baby at feeding time. Being held gives your baby a sense of security that does not come from a propped bottle. If baby vomits or chokes, you will be there to help. Let Dad or other family members share the joy of holding and cuddling the baby while he or she is being fed.

A MENU FOR BABIES

Optimal choice	Breast milk	
Good choice	Commercial formulas; type prescribed by doctor	Many good ones are available, including a number of special-purpose formulas. Most have vitamins and minerals added so supplements are not necessary, except possibly fluoride. Virtually all bottle-fed babies should receive iron-fortified formula (38).
At 1 year	Fresh whole cow milk	For the child *under* age 1, fresh cow milk is hard to digest and is poorly used. It can cause intestinal bleeding, leading to anemia.
Not acceptable	1% or 2% milk, skim milk	Does not provide adequate fat or essential fatty acids. Fat is necessary early in life for brain and nervous-system development. These forms of milk should not be used during the first 24 months of life.

BREAST OR BOTTLE? A SUMMARY

Reasons for Breast-Feeding

- Breast milk is the nutritionally superior food for human babies.
- Breast milk is easily absorbed and digested by infants. Breast-fed babies have less constipation and diarrhea and fewer upsets and allergies.
- Babies who are breast-fed are protected against illness by special disease-fighting antibodies in the mother's milk.
- Nursing utilizes the mother's fat reserves to make milk, helps control postdelivery bleeding, and encourages the return of the uterus to normal size without the use of medication.
- Breast milk is always ready for the baby—clean and fresh.
- Nursing promotes bonding between mother and baby.
- Breast-feeding prevents overfeeding because the baby stops when full.
- Breast-feeding is less expensive than formula.
- Breast-feeding eliminates the need for bottles, bottle washing, and carrying bottles around.

Reasons for Bottle-Feeding

- Some women may find the idea of nursing distasteful.
- Nursing may not be acceptable by the mother's mate or by others whose support she values.
- The mother's work or lifestyle may not allow her the time or conditions required to nurse or express milk.

- A woman may have had a previous unpleasant experience with nursing.
- The father, older children, and caregivers can share in feeding the infant.
- The mother can be more independent.
- Women receiving certain medications may be advised against nursing.
- Women who are HIV positive should not breast-feed.
- Special-purpose formulas may be necessary for babies with particular needs related to health problems.

If you're still undecided, we encourage you to give breastfeeding a try. Commit to a long enough period for nursing to become established—at least six or eight weeks. Then, if you wish, you can either combine breast- and bottle-feeding or wean your baby to formula.

Throughout pregnancy and after your baby is born, you have a responsibility and an opportunity to select healthful foods, avoid harmful substances, and participate in physical activities that will make your child the very best he or she can be. We hope that this book will encourage you and help you make intelligent, informed health and nutrition decisions that will benefit both you and your child.

Answers to Quick Quizzes

Chapter 4. The Proteins, Carbohydrates, and Fats of Pregnancy

1. False
2. False
3. True
4. False
5. True
6. False
7. False
8. True
9. False
10. False

Chapter 5. Mighty Vitamins

1. d. Green pepper
2. c. Vitamin D
3. b. Vitamin A
4. a. Vitamin D
5. d. Folate
6. False
7. False
8. True
9. True
10. False

Chapter 6. Minerals: The Strong Supports

1. Vitamin D
2. Iron
3. Fluoride
4. Iron
5. Chloride
6. False
7. True
8. False
9. True
10. False

Chapter 7. Playing It Safe

1. True
2. True
3. False
4. False
5. False
6. True
7. False
8. True
9. True
10. True

Bibliography

1. *Alphabet Soup: Nutrients from Food and Supplements.* Chicago: The American Dietetic Association, 1987.
2. American Academy of Pediatrics Committee on Psychosocial Aspects of Child and Family Health. "The Mother Working Outside the Home." *Pediatrics* 73 (1984): 874.
3. American College of Obstetricians and Gynecologists. *Exercise During Pregnancy and the Postnatal Period.* Washington, DC: ACOG, 1985.
4. ———. "Guidelines on Pregnancy and Work." Chicago: ACOG, 1987.
5. American College of Obstetricians and Gynecologists and American Dietetic Association. *Assessment of Maternal Nutrition.* Chicago: The American Dietetic Association, 1978.
6. American Council on Science and Health. *The Effects of Caffeine: A Report of the American Council on Science and Health.* Summit, NJ: ACSH, 1981.
7. American Diabetes Association, Inc. *Diabetes in the Family.* Bowie, MD: Robert J. Brady Co., Prentice-Hall Publishing, 1982.
8. American Dietetic Association. "Diet in Pregnancy." In *Manual of Clinical Dietetics.* Chicago: The American Dietetic Association, 1988.
9. Anderson, Garland D. "Clinical Implications of Recent Basic Research in Prenatal Patients." In *Nutrition in Pregnancy,* ed. Emery A. Wilson. Lexington: U. of Kentucky, 1980.

10. Annis, Linda F. *The Child Before Birth.* Ithaca, NY: Cornell University Press, 1978.
11. Bayle, Louise Thompson, and Marcia Butman, eds. *Prenatal Nutrition: A Clinical Manual.* Boston: Massachusetts Department of Public Health, 1989.
12. Beal, Virginia A. "Nutritional Studies During Pregnancy II—Dietary Intake, Maternal Weight Gain, and Infant Size." *Journal of the American Dietetic Association* 58: 321–26.
13. Belizan, J. M., J. Villar, and J. Repke. "The Relationship Between Calcium Intake and Pregnancy-Induced Hypertension: Up-to-Date Evidence." *American Journal of Obstetrics and Gynecology* 158 (1988): 898–902.
14. Berkowitz, Gertrude, M. L. Skovron, R. H. Lapinski, and R. L. Berkowitz. "Delayed Childbearing and the Outcome of Pregnancy." *New England Journal of Medicine* 322 (10) March 8, 1990: pp. 659–64.
15. Bible. Judges 13:4, 13:7.
16. Bracken, M. B., et al. "Coffee Consumption During Pregnancy." *New England Journal of Medicine* 306 (1982): 1548–49.
17. Brezezinski, A., Y. M. Bromberg, and K. Braun. "Riboflavin Deficiency in Pregnancy, Its Relationship to Course of Pregnancy and to Condition of Fetus." *Journal of Obstetrics and Gynecology of the British Empire,* 54 (1947): 182.
18. Briggs, Gerald G., Roger K. Freeman, and J. Sumner. *Drugs in Pregnancy and Lactation: A Reference Guide to Fetal and Neonatal Risk.* 3rd ed. Baltimore: Williams and Wilkins, 1990.
19. Bronstein, E. S., and J. Dollar. "Pica in Pregnancy." *Journal of the Medical Association of Georgia* 63 (1974): 332.
20. Brooke, O. G., et al. "Vitamin D Supplements in Pregnant Asian Women: Effects of Calcium Status and Fetal Growth." *British Medical Journal* 1 (1980): 751.
21. Brown, Judith E., and R. B. Toma. "Taste Changes During Pregnancy." *American Journal of Clinical Nutrition* 43 (1986): 414.

22. "The Bubbly and the Still Rate on the Waterline." *Tribune* (Chicago) 12 Oct. 1983: 7C.
23. Bull, Patricia L. (The Breastfeeding Connection.) Telephone interview. 14 Aug. 1990.
24. Burros, Marian. "Not All the Alcohol Boils Away During Cooking Process." *Tribune* (Chicago) 26 July 1990: Food Guide, 2.
25. Burt, B. A., S. A. Eklund, and W. J. Loesche, "Dental Benefits of Limited Exposure and Fluoridated Water in Childhood." *Journal of Dental Research* 65 (1986): 1322–25.
26. *Caring for Our Future: The Content of Prenatal Care.* A Report of the Public Health Service Expert Panel on the Content of Prenatal Care. Washington, DC: Department of Health and Human Services, 1989.
27. Chaney, N. E., J. Franke, and W. B. Wadlington. "Cocaine Convulsions in a Breast-Feeding Baby." *Journal of Pediatrics* 112 (1988): 134.
28. Chasnoff, Ira J., D. E. Lewis, and L. Squires. "Cocaine Intoxication in a Breast-Fed Infant." *Pediatrics* 80 (1987): 836.
29. Chasnoff, Ira, and S. MacGregor. "Maternal Cocaine Use and Neonatal Morbidity." *Pediatric Research* 21 (1987): 356A.
30. Chesley, L. C. "Blood Pressure, Edema, and Proteinuria in Pregnancy: Historical Developments." *Prog. Clinical Biological Research* 7 (1976): 19–66.
31. Clarren, S. K., et al. "Brain Malformations Related to Prenatal Exposure to Ethanol." *Journal of Pediatrics* 92 (1978): 64–67.
32. Clemens, T. L., et al. "Increased Skin Pigment Reduces the Capacity of Skin to Synthesize Vitamin D_3." *Lancet* 1 (1982): 74–76.
33. Coetzee, E. J., W. P. U. Jackson, and P. A. Berman. "Ketonuria in Pregnancy with Special Reference to Caloric-

Restricted Food Intake in Obese Diabetics." *Diabetes* 29 (1980): 177.

34. Coltman, C. A. "Pagophagia and Iron Lack." *Journal of the American Medical Association* 207 (1969): 513.

35. Committee on Adolescence. "Adolescent Pregnancy." *Pediatrics* 83.1 (1989): 133.

36. Committee on Diet and Health National Research Council. *Diet and Health.* Washington, DC: National Academy Press, 1989.

37. Committee on Nutrition, American Academy of Pediatrics. "Fluoride Supplementation." *Pediatrics* 77 (1986): 758.

38. ———. "Iron-Fortified Infant Formulas." *Pediatrics* 84.6 (1989): 1114.

39. "Contaminated Raw Seafood." *Nutrition & the M.D.* 16.6 (1990): 1.

40. Cornacchia, Harold J., and Stephen Barrett. *Consumer Health: A Guide to Intelligent Decisions.* 2nd ed. St. Louis: Mosby, 1980.

41. Coustan, Donald R., and Sheila Garvey. *The Baby Team.* St. Louis: Monoject Division, Sherwood Medical, 1979.

42. Dalton, K., and M. J. T. Dalton. "Characteristics of Pyridoxine Overdose Neuropathy Syndrome." *Acta. Neurol. Scand.* 76 (1987): 8–11.

43. Dawson, E. B., J. Albears, and W. J. McGanity. "Serum Zinc Changes Due to Iron Supplementation in Teenage Pregnancy." *American Journal of Clinical Nutrition* 50 (1989): 848–52.

44. Dawson-Hughes, Bess, et al. "A Controlled Trial of the Effect of Calcium Supplementation on Bone Density in Postmenopausal Women." *New England Journal of Medicine* 323 (1990): 878–88.

45. Duncan, B., et al. "Iron and the Exclusively Breast-Fed Infant from Birth to Six Months." *Journal of Pediatric Gastroenterology* 4 (1985): 421.

46. Edidin, Deborah V., M.D. "Resurgence of Nutritional Rickets Associated with Breast-Feeding and Special Dietary Practices." *Pediatrics* 6 (1980): 232–35.

47. Eisenberg, Arlene, Heidi E. Murkoff, and Sandee E. Hathaway. *What to Expect When You're Expecting.* New York: Workman, 1984.

48. Enig, Mary G. "Pharmacologic Basis of Drug-Nutrient Interaction Related to Drug Abuse During Pregnancy." *Clinical Nutrition* 6 (6) (1987): 235–43.

49. Ereman, R. R., B. Lonnerdal, and K. G. Dewey. "Maternal Sodium Intake Does Not Affect Postprandial Sodium Concentrations in Human Milk." *Journal of Nutrition* 117 (1987): 1154.

50. Ernhart, C. B., et al. "Alcohol Teratogeneticity in the Human: A Detailed Assessment of Specificity, Critical Period, and Threshold." *American Journal of Obstetrics and Gynecology* 156 (1987): 33.

51. "Even Moderate Drinking May Be Hazardous to Maturing Fetus." *Journal of the American Medical Association* 237 (1977): 2535–36.

52. Fairweather, D. V. I. "Nausea and Vomiting in Pregnancy." *American Journal of Obstetrics and Gynecology* 102 (1968): 135.

53. Farley, Dixie. "Food Safety Crucial for People with Lowered Immunity." Quote from Peter Howley, M. D., Medical Director, Whetman-Walker Clinic, Washington, DC. *FDA Consumer* (July-Aug. 1990): 7–9.

54. Ferguson, B. B., D. S. Wilson, and W. Schaffner. "Determinations of Nicotine Concentrations in Human Milk. *American Journal of Diseases of Children* 130 (1976): 837.

55. Figoletto, F. D., and G. A. Little, eds. *Guidelines for Prenatal Care.* 2nd ed. Washington, DC: American College of Pediatrics and the American College of Obstetricians and Gynecologists, 1988.

56. Filer, Lloyd J., Jr. "Maternal Nutrition and Lactation." *Clinics in Perinatology* 2 (1975): 353–60.

57. Finnegan, Loretta P. "Effects of Caffeine and Nicotine." *Symposia Reporter* 4 (1981): 20–21.

58. "Fluoride Compounds." *Accepted Dental Therapeutics.* 40th ed. Chicago: American Dental Association, 1984, 395–420.

59. Folkenberg, Judy. "Mal de Mere: Simple Remedies Best for Morning Sickness." *FDA Consumer* (Nov. 1988): 26–29.

60. Foltin, R. W., et al. "Marijuana and Cocaine Interactions in Humans: Cardiovascular Consequences." *Pharmacol. Biochem. Behav.* 28 (1987): 459–64.

61. Fomon, S. J., et al. "Excretion of Fat by Normal Full-Term Infants Fed Various Milks and Formulas." *American Journal of Clinical Nutrition* 23 (1970): 1299.

62. *Foodborne Illness in the Home: How and Why What You Eat Can Make You Sick.* Chicago: The American Dietetic Association, 1988.

63. Fox, H. M. "Pantothenic Acid." In *Handbook of Vitamins: Nutritional, Biochemical, and Clinical Aspects,* ed. L. J. Machlin. New York: Marcel Dekker, 1984, 437–57.

64. Frank, Deborah A., et al. "Cocaine Use During Pregnancy: Prevalence and Correlates." *Pediatrics* 82 (6) (1988): 888–95.

65. Frassinelli-Gunderson, E. P., S. Margen, and J. R. Brown. "Iron Stores in Users of Oral Contraceptives Agents." *American Journal of Clinical Nutrition* 41 (1985): 703–12.

66. Fregly, M. J. "Attempts to Estimate Sodium Intake in Humans." In *NIH Workshop on Nutrition and Hypertension,* ed. M. J. Horan, et al. Proceedings of a Symposium, 12–14 Mar.

1984. Bethesda, MD. New York: Biomedical Information Corp., 1985.

67. Freidman, W. F., and L. F. Mills. "The Relationship Between Vitamin D and the Craniofacial and Dental Anomalities of the Supravalvular Aortic Stenosis Syndrome." *Pediatrics* 43 (1969): 12.
68. Freinkel, Norbert. "Summary and Recommendations of the Second International Workshop: Conference on Gestational Diabetes Mellitus." *Diabetes* 34 (Suppl. 2) (1985): 123–26.
69. Freinkel, Norbert, S. L. Dooley, and Boyd E. Metzger. "Care of the Pregnant Woman with Insulin-Dependent Diabetes Mellitus." *New England Journal of Medicine* 313 (1985): 96–101.
70. Fuhrmann, K., et al. "Prevention of Congenital Malformations in Infants of Insulin-Dependent Diabetic Mothers." *Diabetes Care* 6 (1983): 219–23.
71. Gantz, Herb. "An Interview with Dr. Gregory Parham." *Food News for Consumers* 7.2 (1990): 10–11.
72. Glenn, F. B., W. D. Glenn, and R. C. Duncan. "Fluoride Tablet Supplementation During Pregnancy for Caries Immunity: A Study of Offspring Produced." *American Journal of Obstetrics and Gynecology* 143 (1982): 560.
73. Goldfarb, Johanna, and Edith Tibbetts. *Breastfeeding Handbook: A Practical Reference for Physicians, Nurses, and Other Health Professionals.* Hillside, NJ: Enslow Publishers, 1980.
74. Greer, F. R., et al. "Bone Mineral Content and Serum 25-Hydroxyvitamin D Concentrations in Breast-Fed Infants with and Without Supplemental Vitamin D: One Year Follow Up." *Journal of Pediatrics* 100 (1982): 919.
75. Hadeed, Anthony, and Sharon Siegel. "Maternal Cocaine Use During Pregnancy: Effects on the Newborn Infant." *Pediatrics* 84 (2) (1989): 205–10.
76. Hambidge, K. M., and A. M. Mauer. "Trace Elements." Laboratory Indices of Nutritional Status in Pregnancy. *Report*

of the Committee of Nutrition of the Mother and Preschool Child. Washington, DC: Food and Nutrition Board, National Academy of Sciences 1978, 157–93.

77. Hammar, M., et al. "Calcium and Magnesium Status of Pregnant Women. A Comparison Between Treatment with Calcium and Vitamin C in Pregnant Women with Leg Cramps." *International Journal of Vitamin Nutrition Research* 57 (1987): 179–83.
78. Hands, Elizabeth S. *Food Finder: Food Sources of Vitamins and Minerals.* 2nd ed. Salem: ESHA Research, 1990.
79. Heaney, Robert P., et al. "Meal Effects on Calcium Absorption." *American Journal of Clinical Nutrition* 49 (1989): 372–76.
80. Heaney, Robert P., and T. G. Skillman. "Calcium Metabolism in Normal Human Pregnancy." *Journal of Clinical Endocrinology Metabolism* 33 (1971): 661–70.
81. "Heartburn: Why It Occurs, and Ways to Gain Relief." *Environmental Nutrition* (June 1988): 2.
82. Hecht, Annabel. "Advice on Breast-Feeding and Drugs." FDA Consumer 13 (Nov. 1979); HEW Publication No. (FDA)80-3098. U.S. Dept. of Health, Education and Welfare, Public Health Service, Food and Drug Administration, Office of Public Affairs.
83. Heller, S., R. M. Salkeld, and W. F. Korner. "Vitamin B_1 Status in Pregnancy." *American Journal of Clinical Nutrition* 27 (1974): 1221.
84. Henry, Ann Karen, and Jil Feldhausen. *Drugs, Vitamins, Minerals in Pregnancy.* Tucson: Fisher Books, 1989.
85. Hess, Mary Abbott, and Anne Elise Hunt. *Pickles & Ice Cream: The Complete Guide to Nutrition During Pregnancy.* New York: McGraw-Hill, 1982.
86. Hess, Mary Abbott, and Katharine Middleton. *The Art of Cooking for the Diabetic.* Chicago: Contemporary Books, 1988.

87. Hesser, L. "Tartrazine on Trial." *Food Chemical Toxicology* 22 (1984): 1019–24.
88. Hibbard, Roberta A., and Ronald Blevins. "Palatal Burn Due to Bottle Warming in a Microwave Oven." *Pediatrics* 83 (2) (1988): 382–84.
89. Higgins, Agnes. Lecture to the Society for Nutrition Education. Montreal, Quebec, 8 July 1980.
90. Hillman, R. V., et al. "Pyridoxine Supplementation During Pregnancy, Clinical and Laboratory Observations." *American Journal of Clinical Nutrition* 12 (1963): 427.
91. Hinds, Michael deCourcy. "Bottled Water a Health Aid? U.S. and Industry Agree: NO." *New York Times* 13 Aug. 1981.
92. Huggins, Kathleen. *The Nursing Mother's Companion.* Boston: Harvard Common Press, 1986.
93. Hurley, Lucille S. *Developmental Nutrition.* Englewood Cliffs: Prentice-Hall, Inc., 1980.
94. Iber, Frank L. "Fetal Alcohol Syndrome." *Nutrition Today* (Sept.-Oct. 1980): 4–11.
95. Immerman, A. M. "Vitamin B_{12} Status on a Vegetarian Diet." *World Review of Nutrition and Dietetics* 34 (1981): 38–54.
96. Institute of Medicine, Committee to Study the Prevention of Low Birthweight. *Preventing Low Birthweight.* Washington, DC: National Academy Press, 1985.
97. *Iron and Human Nutrition.* Chicago: National Live Stock and Meat Board, 1990.
98. Jones, C. L., and R. E. Lopez. "Direct and Indirect Effects on the Infant of Maternal Drug Abuse." *Report on the Content of Prenatal Care: Background Papers.* Washington, DC: U.S. Public Health Service, 1990.
99. Kaminetzky, Harold A., and Herman Baker. "Micronutrients in Pregnancy. *Clinical Obstetrics and Gynecology* 20 (1977): 363–79.
100. Khaw, K. T., and E. Barrett-Conner. "Dietary Potassium and Stroke-Associated Mortality. A 12-Year Prospective

Population Study." *New England Journal of Medicine* 316 (1987): 235–40.

101. Kiilholma, P., et al. "The Role of Calcium, Copper, Iron, and Zinc in Preterm Delivery and Premature Rupture of Fetal Membranes." *Gynecol. Obstet. Invest.* 17 (1984): 194–201.

102. Kirkinen, P., et al. "The Effect of Caffeine on Placental and Fetal Blood Flow in Human Pregnancy." *American Journal of Obstetrics and Gynecology* 147 (1983): 939–42.

103. Kramer, M. S. "Intrauterine Growth and Gestational Duration Determinants." *Pediatrics* 80 (1987): 502–11.

104. Kumar, S. "Effect of Zinc Supplementation on Rats During Pregnancy." *Nutr. Rep. Int.* 13 (1976): 33–36.

105. Lammer, E. J., et al. "Retinoic Acid Embryopathy." *New England Journal of Medicine,* 313 (1985): 837–41.

106. Lammi-Keefe, C. J., and R. G. Jensen. "Lipids in Human Milk: A Review." *Pediatric Gastroenterology Nutrition* 3 (1984): 172–98.

107. Langford, H. G. "Dietary Potassium and Hypertension." In *NIH Workshop on Nutrition and Hypertension: Proceedings from a Symposium,* ed. M. J. Horan, et al. New York: Biomedical Information Corp., 1985, 147–53.

108. Lawrence, Ruth A. *Breastfeeding: A Guide for the Medical Profession.* 3rd ed. St. Louis: Mosby, 1989.

109. Leathem, A. M. "Safety and Efficacy of Antiemetics Used to Treat Nausea and Vomiting in Pregnancy." *Clinical Pharmacology* 5 (1986): 660–68.

110. Lecos, Chris. "Caution Light on Caffeine." *FDA Consumer* 14 (Oct. 1980): 69.

111. Life Science Research Office (LSRO). *Evaluation of the Health Aspects of Vitamin B_{12} as a Food Ingredient.* Bethesda: Federation of American Society for Experimental Biology, 1978.

112. Little, R. E., and C. F. Sing. "Association of Father's Drinking and Infants' Birth Weight." *New England Journal of Medicine* 314 (1986): 1644.

113. Little, R. E., K. W. Anderson, C. H. Ervin, B. Worthington-Roberts, and S. K. Clarren. "Maternal Alcohol Use During Breast-Feeding and Infant Mental and Motor Development at One Year." *New England Journal of Medicine* 312 (1989): 425–30.

114. Luke, Barbara. "Understanding Pica in Pregnant Women." *The Journal of Maternal Child Nursing* 2 (1977): 97.

115. March of Dimes Birth Defects Foundation. "D*A*T*A*: Drugs, Alcohol, Tobacco Abuse During Pregnancy." White Plains, NY: March of Dimes, 1980.

116. ———. "Pregnancy over 35." White Plains, NY: March of Dimes, 1988.

117. Massey, L. K., and P. W. Hollingbery. "Acute Effects of Dietary Caffeine and Aspirin on Urinary Mineral Excretion in Pre- and Postmenopausal Women." *Nutrition Research* 8 (1988): 845–51.

118. Mayer, Jean, and Jeanne P. Goldberg. *Dr. Jean Mayer's Diet and Nutrition Guide.* New York: Pharos Books, 1990.

119. Meier, Jeff. Telephone interview. 9 Aug. 1990.

120. Mellies, M. J., et al. "The Substitution of Sucrose Polyester for Dietary Fat in Obese, Hypercholesterolemic Outpatients." *American Journal of Clinical Nutrition* 41 (1985): 1–12.

121. Miller, R. K., et al. "Position Paper by the Teratology Society: Vitamin A During Pregnancy." *Teratology* (1987): 267–75.

122. Mills, J. L., et al. "Maternal Alcohol Consumption and Birth Weight. How Much Drinking During Pregnancy Is Safe?" *Journal of the American Medical Association* 252 (1984): 1875–79.

123. Milunsky, Aubrey, et al. "Multivitamin/Folic Acid Supplementation in Early Pregnancy Reduces the Prevalence of Neural Tube Defects." *Journal of the American Medical Association* 262 (1989): 2847–52.

124. Morck, T. A., S. R. Lynch, and J. D. Cook. "Inhibition of Food Iron Absorption by Coffee." *American Journal of Clinical Nutrition* 37 (1983): 416–20.

125. Moser, P. B., and R. D. Reynolds. "Dietary Zinc and Zinc Concentrations of Plasma, Erythrocytes, and Breast Milk in Antepartum and Postpartum Lactating and Nonlactating Women: A Longitudinal Study." *American Journal of Clinical Nutrition* 33 (1980): 198.

126. Munoz, Leda M., B. Lonnerdal, C. L. Keen, and K. G. Dewey. "Coffee Consumption as a Factor in Iron Deficiency Anemia among Pregnant Women and Their Infants in Costa Rica." *American Journal of Clinical Nutrition* 48 (1988): 645–51.

127. Naeye, R. L. "Nutritional-Nonnutritional Interactions that Affect the Outcome of Pregnancy." *American Journal of Clinical Nutrition* 34 (1981): 727–31.

128. Naeye, R. L., and E. C. Peters. "Mental Development of Children Whose Mothers Smoked During Pregnancy." *Obstetrics and Gynecology* 64 (1984): 601–7.

129. National Academy of Sciences. *Maternal Nutrition and the Course of Pregnancy: Report of the Committee on Maternal Nutrition.* Washington, DC: National Research Council, 1970.

130. National Restaurant Association. *1990 National Restaurant Association Food Service Industry Forecast.* Washington, DC: NRA, 1990.

131. Neifert, Dr. Marianne. Lecture at the International Conference of the La Leche League. Chicago, IL, 24 July 1981.

132. Ney, D. M., et al. *The Low Oxalate Diet Book.* San Diego: U. of California, 1981.

133. Oakley, Ray. *Drugs, Society, and Human Behavior.* 2nd ed. St. Louis: Mosby, 1978.

134. Opp, Marcia. "Back to the Breast." *Family Style* 1 (1981): 20.

135. Pennington, Jean A. T., ed. *Food Values of Portions Commonly Used.* 15th ed. New York: Harper, 1989.

136. Pennington, J. A. T., B. E. Young, and D. B. Wilson. "Nutritional Elements in U.S. Diets: Results from the Total Diet Study, 1982–1986." *Journal of the American Dietetic Association* 89 (1989): 659–64.

137. Phillips, Margaret C., and George M. Briggs. "Symposium: Milk and Dairy Products for the American Diet." *Journal of Dairy Science* 58 (1975): 1751–63.

138. Picciano, Mary Frances. Presentation to Institute of Food Technologists, Chicago Chapter, Rosemont, IL, 16 April 1990.

139. Picone, T. A., et al. "Pregnancy Outcome in North American Women. I. Effects of Diet, Cigarette Smoking, and Psychological Stress on Maternal Weight Gain." *American Journal of Clinical Nutrition* 36 (1982): 1205.

140. Pierson, R. N., et al. "Aspirin and Gastrointestinal Bleeding: Chromate 51 Blood Loss Studies. *American Journal of Medicine* 31 (1961): 259–65.

141. Pitkin, Roy M. "Nutritional Support in Obstetrics and Gynecology." *Clinical Obstetrics and Gynecology* 19 (1976): 489–513.

142. "Position of the American Dietetic Association: Vegetarian Diets." Technical Support Paper. *Journal of the American Dietetic Association* 88 (1988): 352.

143. Powers, Margaret A. *Handbook of Diabetes Nutritional Management.* Rockville, MD: Aspen Publications, 1987.

144. "Pregnancy and Alcohol Warning." *FDA Consumer* 15 (8): 2.

145. "A Primer on Dietary Minerals." *FDA Consumer,* (Sept, 1974): In *HEW Publication No. FDA 77-2070.* Washington, DC: HEW, 77–2070.

146. Pritchard, J. A., et al. "Blood Volume Changes in Pregnancy and the Puerperium. II. Red Blood Cell Loss and Changes in Apparent Blood Volume During and Following Vaginal Delivery, Cesarian Section, and Cesarian Section Plus Total Hysterectomy." *American Journal of Obstetrics and Gynecology* 84 (1962): 1271–82.

147. Pryor, Karen. *Nursing Your Baby.* New York: Harper & Row, 1973.

148. Raphael, Dana. *The Tender Gift: Breast-Feeding.* New York: Schocken Books, 1976.

149. "Recommendations Concerning Supplement Usage: ADA Statement." *Journal of the American Dietetic Association* 87 (1987): 1342.

150. Rodman, H. M., et al. "Diabetic Retinopathy and Its Relationship to Pregnancy. In *The Diabetic Pregnancy: A Perinatal Perspective,* eds. I. R. Mercatz and P. J. Adams. New York: Grune and Stratton, 1979, 73–91.

151. Romney, S. L., ed. *Gynecology and Obstetrics: The Healthcare of Women,* 2nd ed. New York: McGraw-Hill, 1981.

152. *Ross Laboratories Mother's Survey.* Columbus, OH: Ross Laboratories, 1987.

153. Rush, D., et al. "The National WIC Evaluation: Evaluation of the Special Supplemental Food Program for Women, Infants, and Children. V. Longitudinal Study of Pregnant Women." *American Journal of Clinical Nutrition* 48 (1988): 439–83.

154. Ryan, Alan S., and Gilbert A. Martinez. "Breast-Feeding and the Working Mother: A Profile." *Pediatrics* 83 (4) (1989): 524–31.

155. *Safe at the Plate: Additives in Food.* Chicago: The American Dietetic Association, 1989.

156. *Safe Keeping for Safe Eating: Tips on Proper Food Storage.* Chicago: The American Dietetic Association, 1988.

157. Sandstrom B., et al. "Oral Iron, Dietary Ligands, and Zinc Absorption." *Journal of Nutrition* 115 (1985): 411–14.

158. Satter, Ellyn. *Child of Mine.* Palo Alto, CA: Bull Publishing, 1986.

159. Scheier, Julie, R.D. Telephone interview. 10 Aug. 1990.

160. Schuster, K., L. B. Bailey, and C. S. Mahan. "Lack of Relationship Between Vitamin B_6 Status and Degree of Morning Sickness in Pregnancy." *Federation Proceedings* 42 (1983): 553.

161. Schwartz, R., B. J. Apgar, and E. M. Wein. "Apparent Absorption and Retention of Ca, Cu, Mg, Mn, and Zn from a Diet Containing Bran." *American Journal of Clinical Nutrition* 43 (1986): 444–55.

162. Secretary's Task Force on Black and Minority Health. *Black and Minority Health.* Washington, DC: U.S. Department of Health and Human Services, 1985.

163. Shajania, A. M., G. Harnaday, and P. H. Barnes. "Oral Contraceptives and Folate Metabolism." *Lancet* 1 (1969): 886.

164. Simko, Margaret D., Catherine Cowell, and Maureen S. Hreha. *Practical Nutrition: A Quick Reference Guide for the Health Care Practitioner.* Rockville, MD: Aspen Publishers, 1989.

165. Simon, T. L., P. J. Garry, and E. M. Hooper. "Iron Stores from Blood Donors." *Journal of the American Medical Association* 245 (1981): 2038–43.

166. Sklar, R. "Nutritional Vitamin B_{12} Deficiency in a Breast-Fed Infant of a Vegan-Diet Mother." *Clinical Pediatrics* 25 (1986): 219–21.

167. Smithells, R. W., S. Sheppard, and C. J. Schorah. "Vitamin Deficiencies and Neural Tube Defects." *Archives Diseases of Children* 51 (1976): 944.

168. Sonstegard, Lois. "Pregnancy-Induced Hypertension: Prenatal Nursing Concerns." *American Journal of Maternal Child Nursing* 4 (1979): 90–95.
169. Srisuphan, W., and M. B. Bracken. "Caffeine Consumption During Pregnancy and Association with Late Spontaneous Abortion." *American Journal of Obstetrics and Gynecology* 154 (1986): 14–20.
170. Stehlin, Doris. "Lactation Suppression Safer Without Drugs." *FDA Consumer* 24 (3): 25–27.
171. Sturtevant, F. M. "Use of Aspartame in Pregnancy." *International Journal of Fertility* 30 (1985): 850.
172. Subcommittee on Nutritional Status and Weight Gain During Pregnancy, et al. *Nutrition During Pregnancy.* Washington, DC: National Academy Press, 1990.
173. Subcommittee on Nutritional Status During Lactation, et al. *Nutrition During Lactation,* Washington, DC: National Academy Press, 1991.
174. Subcommittee on the Tenth Edition of the RDAs, Food and Nutrition Board, Commission of Life Sciences, and National Research Council. *Recommended Dietary Allowances.* 10th ed. Washington, DC: National Academy Press, 1989.
175. "Surgeon General's Advisory on Alcohol and Pregnancy." *FDA Drug Bulletin* 11 (July 1981).
176. *Surgeon General's Workshop on Breast-Feeding and Human Lactation.* Pub. HRS-D-MC-8-2. Washington, DC: Department of Health and Human Services, 1984.
177. Taylor, Flora. "Aspirin: America's Favorite Drug." *FDA Consumer* 14 (Dec. 1980.–Jan. 1981): 12–16.
178. Thomas, M. Rita, and Georgia L. Baker. "Letters to the Editor." *Journal of the American College of Nutrition* 7 (4) (1988): 325–29.
179. Tierson, F. D., C. L. Olsen, and E. B. Hook. "Nausea and Vomiting of Pregnancy and Association with Pregnancy Out-

come." *American Journal of Obstetrics and Gynecology* 155 (1986): 1017–22.

180. Toenjes, Tracy. Telephone interview. 9 Aug. 1990.

181. Tompkins, Winslow T., D. G. Weihl, and R. Mitchell. "The Underweight Patient as an Increased Obstetric Hazard." *American Journal of Obstetrics and Gynecology* 69 (1955): 114–27.

182. Tripp, J. H., and A. W. McNinch. "Haemorrhagic Disease and Vitamin K." *Archives of Diseases of Children* 62 (1987): 436.

183. U.S. Department of Health, Education, and Welfare, and Public Health Service. *The Health Consequences of Smoking.* Washington, DC: GPO, 1975.

184. ———. *Symposium on Human Lactation.* Washington, DC: GPO, 1976.

185. U.S. Department of Health and Human Services. *The Surgeon General's Report on Nutrition and Health.* Washington, DC: GPO, 1988.

186. U.S. Department of Health and Human Services, Public Health Service Expert Panel on the Content of Prenatal Care. *Caring for Our Future: The Content of Prenatal Care.* Washington, DC: GPO, 1989.

187. Van Thiel, D. H., et al. "Alcohol-Induced Testicular Atrophy: An Experimental Model for Hypogonadism Occurring in Chronic Alcoholic Men." *Gastroenterology* 69 (1975): 326.

188. Villar, J., et al. "Calcium Supplementation Reduces Blood Pressure During Pregnancy: Results of a Randomized Controlled Clinical Trial." *Obstetrics and Gynecology* 70 (1987): 70.

189. Wertz, A. W., et al. "Tryptophan-Niacin Relationships in Pregnancy." *Journal of Nutrition* 64 (1958): 339–53.

190. Wheatley, D. "Treatment of Pregnancy Sickness." *British Journal of Obstetrics and Gynaecology* 84 (1977): 444.

191. Whitehead, R. G. "Nutrition and Lactation." *Postgraduate Medical Journal* 55 (1979): 303–10.
192. Whitney, Eleanor Noss, Corinne Balog Cataldo, and Sharon Rady Rolfes. *Understanding Normal and Clinical Nutrition.* 2nd ed. St. Paul: West Publishing Co., 1987.
193. Wideman, C. L., G. H. Baird, and O. T. Bolding. "Ascorbic Acid Deficiency and Premature Rupture of Fetal Membranes." *American Journal of Obstetrics and Gynecology* 88 (1964): 592.
194. Williams, Sue Rodwell. *Nutrition and Diet Therapy.* 6th ed. St. Louis: Times Mirror/Mosby College Publishing, 1989.
195. Willis, Judith. "New Warnings about Accutane and Birth Defects." *FDA Consumer,* Oct. 1988: 27–29.
196. Winick, Myron. *Nutrition and Pregnancy.* White Plains, NY: March of Dimes, 1986.
197. ———. *Nutrition, Pregnancy, and Early Infancy.* Baltimore: Williams and Wilkins, 1989.
198. Wolf, H. "Hormonal Alterations of Efficiency of Conversion of Tryptophan to Urinary Metabolitics of Niacin in Men." *American Journal of Clinical Nutrition* 24 (1971): 792–99.
199. Woods, J. R., Jr., M. A. Plessinger, and K. E. Clark. "Effect of Cocaine on Uterine Blood Flow and Fetal Oxygenation." *Journal of the American Medical Association* 257 (1987) 10: 957–61.
200. World Health Organization. *Contemporary Patterns of Breast-Feeding. Report on the WHO Collaborative Study on Breast-Feeding.* Geneva: WHO, 1981.
201. Worthington-Roberts, Bonnie, et al. "Dietary Cravings and Aversions in the Postpartum Period." *Journal of the American Dietetic Association* 89 (1989): 647–51.
202. Worthington-Roberts, Bonnie S., Joyce Vermeersch, and Sue Rodwell Williams. *Nutrition in Pregnancy and Lactation.* 4th ed. St. Louis: Times Mirror/Mosby College Publishing, 1989.

203. Wu, Stella. "Understanding Maternal Weight Gain Recommendations." New York State Dietetic Association Annual Meeting, Saratoga Springs, NY, 11 May 1990.

204. Yadrick, Martin K., M. A. Kenney, and Esther A. Winterfeldt. "Iron, Copper, and Zinc Status: Response to Supplementation with Zinc and Iron in Adult Females." *American Journal of Clinical Nutrition* 49 (1989): 145–50.

205. Zuckerman, B., et al. "Effects of Maternal Marijuana and Cocaine Use on Fetal Growth. *New England Journal of Medicine* 320 (1989): 762–68.

Index